I0410591

Safer Medical Care For You and Yours

SIX TOOLS FOR SAFE, EFFECTIVE COMPASSIONATE CARE

T Michael White MD

A HealthCare Value Professional

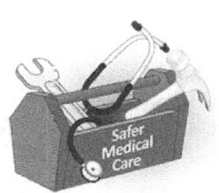 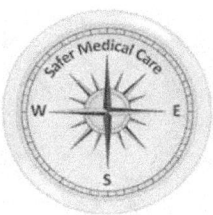 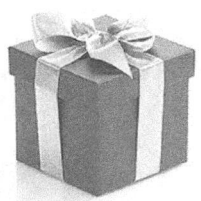

With commentary by geriatric specialist

Stephen F Hightower MD FACP

Copyright © 2016 T Michael White MD All rights reserved.
ISBN: 1539473678
ISBN 13: 9781539473671
Library of Congress Control Number: 2016917915
CreateSpace Independent Publishing Platform
North Charleston, South Carolina

Table of Contents

Dedication

Safer Medical Care for You and Yours — Six Tools for Safe, Effective Compassionate Care is dedicated to the better angels who unfailingly assemble and care for us so well and to us —the involved, informed and responsible who enable their care.

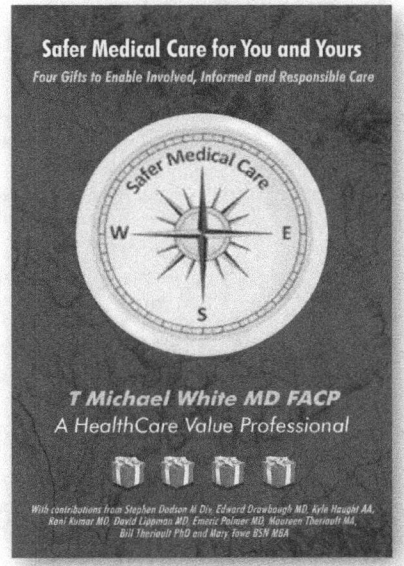

Acknowledgements

wish to recognize and express gratitude to the following individuals for their consideration of my work (the versions above and this undertaking), for their insights and wisdom and for their encouragement: Ms. Maureen Theriault (professional editor and public relations professional), Revered Stephen Dodson and Mr. Matthew Hightower (webmasters), Mr. Kyle Haught (graphic artist), Ms. Terri Hightower and Mr. Colin and Ms. Jackie White (editors), Dr. Ellen Amalfitano and Ms. Mary Towe (nursing leadership and clinical thought leaders), Dr. Ed Drawbaugh (colleague, physician executive, photographer and mentor), Drs. Jim Bernene and Ibrahim Ghobrial (graduate medial education leadership), Dr. Alex Zoretich (medical student perspective) and Dr. Stephen Hightower (warm, wise and encouraging collaborator).

So, What Is In It for You?

f I were to have the honor to sit across from you at your kitchen table, I would convey an important message for you and for those near and dear to you.

The Center for Disease Control estimates there will be over 160 million visits to emergency rooms in 2016. If you also include those who visit an urgent care setting, one out of three of us will seek care in an emergency department or in urgent care in the next year. Although these are excellent institutions, it is very likely they will not have a copy of your medical records, especially if you are visiting from out of town. Without your organized and accurate medical record at your fingertips you will be in a compromised, unsafe position if you should be seriously injured or become significantly ill and lose the capacity to think and speak clearly. I am committed to help you stay safe.

As I have matured as a physician and in life, and as I have begun to address the care of my family (for example, for my well-past 90 mother living large in Florida) and grudgingly confront my own infirmities, I have become a more complete physician. Through training and experience, I have come to understand that we, you and I, are not prepared to enable the fine better angels that assemble to care for us to provide us with safe, effective compassionate care. We, you and I, are not as involved in, informed about and responsible for our healthcare as we should be — as we must be.

What does "involved in, informed about and responsible" for our healthcare look like? It requires that we:

- Craft our organized and accurate uniquely personal medical record and keep it at our fingertips — a major issue;
- Thoughtfully identify and appoint our HealthCare Power of Attorney — a major issue;
- Get in touch with our very personal healthcare values — our wishes for our control of the end of our lives. Then we must commit them to the written page and share them with our HealthCare Power of Attorney — a "major" major issue;
- Learn how to efficiently and effectively convey our medical concerns to our healthcare team;
- Be prepared to, from time to time if/when necessary, to seek the assistance of an advocate who understands how healthcare works and who is invested in your well-being; and
- Keep a prominently displayed emergency alert card on our person with the contact information for our HealthCare Power of Attorney.

How will this help you and yours and me and mine, you might ask? Based upon my training and experience, the reasons are many:

- You will become a much more informed patient;
- Information is power and your healthcare team will be dealing powerfully with information about you;
- Your care will be more efficient making time available for thinking about and caring for you;

- Errors (for example, medications or allergies) will be avoided;
- Expenses (for example, appointments, tests, co-pays and deductibles) will be diminished;
- Your care will feel much more personal and compassionate;
- Your unique and very personal wishes will be honored; and
- Your healthcare team and your significant others will love you for it.

In short, my message for you and for those near and dear to you — become involved in, informed about and responsible for your healthcare. Use the six gift tools provided to enable the better angels assembled to care for you to provide you with safe, effective compassionate care. Start today.

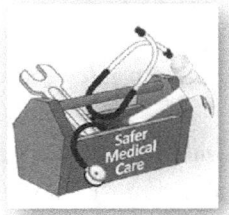

A Charismatic Story: *LaGuardia*

When Einstein was asked about the most powerful force in the universe, he reportedly said, "a charismatic story." To bring the "what's in it for you" to life, let me share a totally fictitious all too true epiphany with you. I call it — *LaGuardia*.

I had just surveyed a fine hospital in Queens for The Joint Commission and was delayed in a surprisingly civilized La Guardia restaurant. I was making the most of a tolerable dinner happily paid for with other people's money. Without provocation a lesion on a prominent part of my face began to profusely bleed. A major farrago, a true debacle ensued. As I set out in search of a bandage, many became flummoxed. It turns out it is not socially acceptable to hemorrhage in public. Who knew? 30 muddled minutes later my snout was most conspicuously, inartistically bandaged. Too tired to be humiliated, I limped onto a much-delayed flight towards home.

On the tarmac, awaiting take-off and anticipating nod-off, reality came to me. I had just experienced a life changing near-miss. If my mortifying but inconsequential bleed had been in my brain rather than on my nose, I would have been brought, without my wits about me, by strangers to a strange Queens' emergency department. There, well-intentioned strange better angels, knowing nothing about me, would assemble to care for me. This panicked me.

Unable to sleep, with purpose I strolled the airplane aisle to scrutinize my fellow travelers. The picture was not a pretty one. Unlike the bullet-proof and invincible travelers they (and I) envision ourselves to be, they were, like me, a weary, vulnerable lot.

This epiphany started me on a mission — to assist you and yours and me and mine to enable safe, effective compassionate care. Disraeli states, "The best way to become acquainted with a subject is to write about it" — so I wrote this book. If there were cliff notes, they might read: just jump to Tool 1: *My (Unique and Very) Personal Medical Record* (page 17); understand it; emulate it; keep it at your fingertips — and don't leave home without it. Then, pass the gift forward by assisting your near and dear to do the same.

If you desire to move forward but find yourself stymied, contact me. I will be pleased to hear from you. I am prepared to efficiently and effectively move you from where you are to where you desire to be. It is what I do.

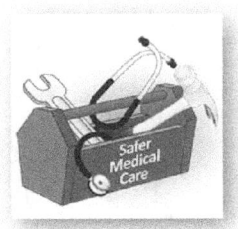

Introduction

The Institute of Medicine has put forward a well-conceived and clearly articulated national goal — for each individual to be provided healthcare that is safe, timely, efficient, effective, equitable (just/fair) and patient-centered (STEEEP). Provided my training and experience, I emphatically concur with and endorse the Institute of Medicine's logic and goal.

The purpose of this concise brochure is to position each unique individual — you, me and those near and dear to us — to enable the better angels assembled to care for us to provide us with safe, effective compassionate care.

This brochure accomplishes this by providing examples of six gift tools for the individual to understand, appreciate and then emulate in her/his uniquely personal manner. The gift tools are as follows:

1. My (Unique and Very) Personal Medical Record
2. My Chief Complaint (my story — why I am here today)
3. My (Unique and Very) Personal HealthCare Values/Wishes
4. My HealthCare Power of Attorney (and My Advanced Directives)
5. My Personal Professional Patient Advocate (My P3A)
6. My Safer Medical Care Emergency Alert System

These tools are gifts to you of the peace and tranquility associated with confidence that your care will be safe and effective and your unique and very personal values and wishes will be honored should complex healthcare circumstances arise.

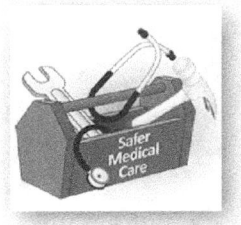

Frequently Asked Questions (FAQs)

An efficient and effective way to "get a feel for" a complex message is to consider the answers to frequently asked questions (FAQs). Answers to some FAQs about *Safer Medical Care for You and Yours— Six Tools for Safe, Effective Compassionate Care* follow:

Q: Why might I read on — what is in it for me?

A: By design, this brief book is all about enhancing the safe, timely, efficient, effective, equitable (fair/just) patient-centered healthcare (some refer to this as STEEEP) provided to you and those near and dear to you. The key is for you to become involved in, informed about and responsible for your healthcare. I anticipate this question and answer session will assist you in understanding why you, with your own very personal circumstances in mind, should start by creating your own *My (Unique and Very) Personal Medical Record*.

Q: Please explain your six gift tools.

A: To realize safer effective, compassionate care, I offer six gift tools:

- Tool 1: *My (Unique and Very) Personal Medical Record — a gift example.* This is an example of a concise organized and accurate personal medical record that, kept at your fingertips, will position you to enable and receive safer medical care.
- Tool 2: *My Chief Complaint (my story — why I am here today) — a gift example.* This tool teaches you how to efficiently and effectively convey your acute (today) healthcare story to your assembled healthcare team so they may do their best for you in your time of need.
- Tool 3: *My (Unique and Very) Personal HealthCare Values/Wishes — a gift example.* This example assists you get in touch with, organize and personalize your very special and unique healthcare wishes so they may be conveyed should complex circumstances require. Many find comfort and peace in this process.
- Tool 4: *My HealthCare Power of Attorney (and My Advanced Directives).* This discussion encourages and assists you to move from the daunting task of addressing complex plans to having your will, your power of attorney, your HealthCare Power of Attorney and your healthcare values/wishes in order.
- Tool 5: *My Personal Professional Patient Advocate (My P3A) — a gift example.* This example describes a special relationship between you and a healthcare savvy individual in your life who, as your personal advocate, is there to assist you and yours navigate complex healthcare circumstances.
- Tool 6: *My Safer Medical Care Emergency Alert System.* This gift tool facilitates notification of your HealthCare Power of Attorney and access to your personal medical record if/when you have lost the capacity to speak for yourself.

Q: Who will benefit from this?

A: Based upon training and experience, I have every confidence:

1. You will. I anticipate you will immediately enable and receive safer, timely, efficient, effective, equitable (fair/just) patient-centered medical care.
2. Your healthcare team will. Your *My (Unique and Very) Personal Medical Record* document will make the work of the best and brightest better angels caring for you more efficient and effective — and they will love you for it.
3. Your family/significant-others — those near and dear to you — will. In complex circumstances, your family/significant-others will be positioned to assist you to receive safe, effective compassionate care and ensure your very personal healthcare values and wishes are honored — and they will love you for it.

Q: Where might I best start?

A: Please start by reviewing and understanding *My (Unique and Very) Personal Medical Record — a gift example* (page 17). Then create your own document (and/or a document for someone near and dear to you) and keep it at your fingertips.

Q: If I invest the time and energy to create My (Unique and Very) Personal Medical Record and have it at my fingertips, how will I be in a better place?

A: Let me count the ways:

1. You will immediately, in a new way, be involved in, informed about and responsible for your healthcare.
2. You will be prepared to efficiently and effectively convey your organized, accurate, legible and up-to date healthcare story to the fine healthcare team assembled to care for you.
3. Your fine healthcare team will efficiently and effectively comprehend your story. You will, to your advantage, convert their work from the inefficient data collection to the invaluable work of thinking about (i.e., diagnosing and treating) you.
4. With your story efficiently and effectively conveyed and comprehended, you have positioned yourself to enable and receive safer, effective compassionate care.
5. With your story efficiently and effectively conveyed and comprehended, you will position your fine healthcare team to accomplish their important, meaningful work and they will love you for it.

Q: Don't my wonderful care givers (my better angels) already have this information?

A: In this day and age, it is unlikely that your healthcare team will have efficient access to your medical information that is organized and accurate.

Q: Doesn't my fine personal physician already have *My (Unique and Very) Personal Medical Record* in order?

A: Perhaps. However, in this day and age, it is wise for you to be prepared for an intricate and vulnerable time when your personal physician will not be involved in your care (for example, while traveling or when referred to a specialist at a major medical center).

Q: Let me ask this same question in a different way. Isn't this information already in my record?

A: There are several "ifs" here:

1. If you have a meticulous, long-term personal physician and if he/she is the only physician who cares for you, the information may be in your record and/or in her/his consciousness;
2. If you have a meticulous, long-term personal physician and see several consultants, your personal physician's record is very likely incomplete and inaccurate;
3. Even if you have a meticulous, long-term personal physician who has your records in perfect order, it is increasingly unlikely that he/she will care for your next acute event. It is more likely you will be cared for by urgent care or emergency medicine staff, by a covering physician, by a hospitalist and/or by a consulted specialist who do not have access to your records and
4. Regrettably, if you were discharged from the hospital just yesterday and re-admitted today to the very same hospital, it is unlikely that your healthcare information in your chart would be organized, accurate and ready to maximally position you to receive safer, timely, efficient, effective, equitable (fair/just) patient-centered medical care.

Q: OK then, let me again ask this same question in a different way. Doesn't my healthcare team assemble this information when I present to the office, urgent care, the emergency department or to the hospital for admission? Isn't that part of standard operating procedure?

A: You may rest assured that the better angels caring for you will in every circumstance do their professional very best, however:

1. The more organized you are, the more organized, efficient, effective and accurate they will be,
2. Caution: you may be in no condition (may not have the capacity) to cooperate with their complex queries and
3. Caution: it will generally take your dedicated and talented team more than an hour to get this right and they often have only minutes — placing your care on the slippery slope just when you most need safer, timely, efficient, effective, equitable (fair/just), medical care.

Q: When I get into this, should I be extremely compulsive about this? Is more, more?

A: Yes and no:

1. Be really compulsive about accuracy (for example, the names and dosages of your medications and at the same time
2. Keep your *My (Unique and Very) Personal Medical Record* to two pages or you will lose your audience — the fine healthcare team assembled to care for you. For your better angels, two organized and accurate pages is best — as is so often the case, less is more.

Q: Why do I (a non-healthcare person) need a *My Personal Professional Patient Advocate (My P3A)*?

A: Based upon experience, when your healthcare becomes complex and you become intricate and vulnerable, it is valuable to have someone close to you who is knowledgeable about healthcare and who has the time to comprehend what is transpiring and patiently translate and frame what is transpiring to you. This positions you to:

1. Be involved in, informed about and responsible for your healthcare,
2. Better cooperate with your care,

3. Make better decisions and
4. Better convey your unique and very personal healthcare values and ensure your wishes are addressed.

Q: What is your motivation Dr. White — what is in it for you?

A: An insightful and fair question. I am on a mission. I fervently and passionately desire to assist you and yours to enable and receive safer, timely, efficient, effective, equitable (fair/just) patient-centered medical care. If, as a public service, I can realize that goal (even if just in a small way), I will recognize important, meaningful work that makes a difference and be handsomely compensated by "a job well done."

Q: What are users saying about this process?

A: Feedback to date:

1. Patients and families/significant-others say they are much more involved in, informed about and responsible for enabling and receiving safer, timely, efficient, effective, equitable (fair/just) patient-centered medical care.
2. Nurses, pharmacists, physicians and staff report finding the two-page *My (Unique and Very) Personal Medical Record* document incredibly useful — especially at first visits, when circumstances become confused and/or after major interventions.
3. Patients and physicians say that the process has helped them identify and address some important neglected healthcare opportunities (for example, catching up on cancer detection, updating immunizations and/or identifying medication incompatibilities).
4. Patients, families/significant-others, physicians and support staff report enhanced communications.
5. Families/significant-others report they find it helpful to assist less computer (word processing) savvy family members/friends with document preparation.
6. Patients, nurses, pharmacists, physicians, staff and families/significant-others have recommended this process to their own family and friends.
7. All observe this is not rocket science — it is just as important as rocket science as it favorably impacts clinical, quality, safety, satisfaction and financial aspects of healthcare.

Q: If this works out for me and mine, how may I repay the favor?

A: Thanks for asking,

1. If you were to create and implement your own *My (Unique and Very) Personal Medical Record* that will be reward enough for me.
2. I would be ecstatic if you were to pass the concept, *My (Unique and Very) Personal Medical Record*, forward to those near and dear to you.
3. *Safer Medical Care for You and Yours* is a continuous quality improvement process. It will assist my work greatly if you were to communicate (drmikewhite@tmichaelwhitemd.com or safermedcare@gmail.com) that which I have right (and why), that which I have wrong (and why) and that which I have missed/omitted.

Again thanks for asking.

Q: What if I have done my best and still have a question or two?

A: This is important. I will be pleased to do my best to answer an email question or two regarding the process of creating your documents — it is what I do. I may best be contacted at drmikewhite@tmichaelwhitemd.com or safermedcare@gmail.com.

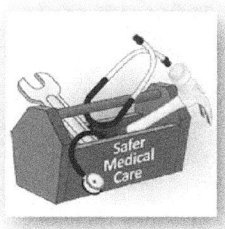

Concise Brochure/Primer

was not sure how to categorize this treatise on *Safer Medical Care for You and Yours*. By intent, with the wise and warm assistance of geriatric specialist Dr. Stephen Hightower, it summarizes a previously published book full of "nice to know," *Safer Medical Care for You and Yours — Four Gifts to Enable Involved, Informed and Responsible Care*, into a concise package of "need to know." So I went to the thesaurus and considered booklet, guide, brochure, etc. Coming upon and exploring the definitions of primer, I thought I would settle on that. From Webster a primer can be:

- A small introductory book on a subject; or
- A charged cap, cylinder, molecule (or idea) that ignites an explosion.

But, I came to realize that primer is very much a British word and I was making the simple complex. So the previous book has been condensed into this brochure — a small book containing information about a product or service.

At the same time, I very much hope *Safer Medical Care for You and Yours — Six Tools for Safe, Effective Compassionate Care* will, like the primer it is, put a charge in you that will ignite change in your life and in the lives of those near and dear to you.

This brochure (and primer) is intentionally concise. By design it is short and sweet and to the point. For a more complete understanding of from where these tools emanate, please peruse my book: *Safer Medical Care for You and Yours — Four Gifts to Enable Involved, Informed and responsible Care* (available at Amazon and Kindle) — a book that patiently provides the background information and stories that have led me to become a passionate advocate for safe, effective compassionate care who feels compelled to place six gift tools at your fingertips.

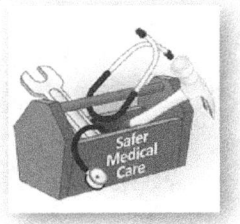

Dr. Stephen Hightower —
A Geriatrician's Perspective

This primer has become a combined effort. By design, I will concisely state a concept and Dr. Stephen Hightower, a distinguished New Mexico geriatrician who guides the care of several thousand patients, will add his insights immediately below my text. His brief bio, along with mine, is included at the end of this brochure.

Dr. Stephen Hightower Comments

As an advocate for Dr. White's advancement of safer, effective and compassionate care, I am delighted to have this opportunity to offer my insights. They come entirely from my training for and my experience with the care of mature patients.

My comments reflect the conversations I have with my patients and their significant others every day. By design, my comments are written and will hopefully read as if I am speaking with an individual patient and family.

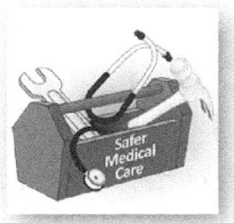

Involved, Informed and Responsible Care — Prevention

My industrial engineering quality guru, the now deceased Dr. Phil Crosby, taught me that quality healthcare requires:

- A **definition** — conformance to mutually agreed upon requirements (for example, done right, on time and within budget);
- A **standard/attitude** — error free care done right the first time;
- A **measurement** — the sobering personal and financial cost of a medical error; and
- A **system** — prevention.

His lessons have held up and served me well. I shall be forever grateful for his sharing his insights with me.

Upfront, Dr. Crosby warns that prevention is the biggest challenge as it is hard work. Prevention requires that we each:

- Become involved in, informed about and responsible for our care;
- Become involved in, informed about and responsible for the care of the near and dear entrusted to us;
- Step away from our way-too-busy day to day — the really hard part; and
- Seriously plan for healthcare circumstances that we (bullet-proof and invincible) are confident will never occur.

Prevention is arduous hard work. This brochure entreats you step up to the task of putting your (and that of the near and dear entrusted to you) organized and accurate healthcare information in order so you may have it at your fingertips if/when you, your family and/or the better angels that care for you need it. More importantly, this primer provides the tools you need to easily accomplish the task.

Dr. Stephen Hightower Comments

You are an amazingly special person in this world. You are valued by family, friends, colleagues and people who have simply had the good fortune to make your acquaintance. Continue your joy, insights, and experiences in this life, but for your sake, and for the sake of those you cherish, take action to be safe. Random events and unforeseen accidents occur too commonly.

Realizing that knowledge is power, become personally prepared by using the six tools outlined in detail in this brochure. When you provide this information to those professionals that step up to help you (Dr. White's better angels) address challenging times, you provide them the power of knowledge about you and you give them their best opportunity to treat you well and maintain you as the amazingly special person you are.

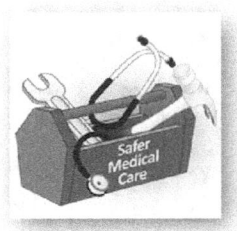

Imagine

magine that you, like me, are a bullet-proof, invincible individual who may take an age-appropriate pill or two but who surely will never require complex medical care. Imagine that the unthinkable happens — while traveling you become quite ill and require unanticipated complex care in an environment strange to you. Let us make it a tad more interesting — because of your unanticipated illness, you are not quite your sharp as a laser, clear-thinking self. Should this happen, the better angels assembled to care for you immediately require: an understanding of what has recently transpired; your chronological medical history; your allergies; your medications; and your HealthCare Power of Attorney contact information.

If this information is at your fingertips, you (an involved, informed and responsible patient) will enable your fine healthcare team to meet the Institute of Medicine's goal — care that is safe, timely, efficient, effective equitable/just and patient-centered (STEEEP). If this information is not available, you have placed yourself (and your healthcare team) on a dangerously slippery healthcare slope. Less obvious but equally important — you have tremendously handicapped and complicated the lives for those closest to you who may have to intercede on your behalf.

Dr. Stephen Hightower Comments

Imagination for most of us contains a positive sense of fulfillment for something we need or desire. These thoughts provoke happiness, comfort and the positive emotions of a good, what if, world. At this time, however, we are asking you to do the hard work of imagining something that is not positive or fulfilling — imagine an unanticipated unfortunate illness, injury, trauma, or perhaps a significant pain or new symptom when you are away from home.

I began my medical practice after residency by working for four years with the Public Health Service in a small New Mexico town of 7,000 called Truth or Consequences — its real name. T or C lies between the largest highway in New Mexico, Interstate-25, and the largest lake in New Mexico, Elephant Butte. It is 80 miles from any other major city. For 6 months of the year, each weekend would see as many as 100,000 people from New Mexico and Texas flocking to enjoy that lake.

Because we had no emergency medicine doctors, my three colleagues and I rotated to cover the emergency room at our 32 bed hospital. This was quite a growth experience for me — I became adept at removing fishing lures from unimaginable body parts. Caring for boating and car accident victims was more challenging.

Back then — and too often today — no one carried any information about themselves. It was like working in the dark. In the midst of crisis, as I established intravenous lines and stabilized blood pressure and breathing, I would struggle to piece together information from semiconscious patients and frightened family members. It was an arduous, imperfect task.

A better understanding of their underlying medical problems, their medications and their allergies would have helped me treat these patients in T or C. By necessity, I became well acquainted with the trauma service at the University of New Mexico and their fine supportive helicopter team. A better understanding of each patient would have helped me prepare them for an effective and efficient handoff to the University trauma team.

The reality is I did not save everybody. I lost both young and old. In my mind, accurate and organized information equates to power — power to advance safe, effective compassionate care.

There are lots of wonderful big and small towns in the United States and in the world worth visiting. There are also many unique experiences to enjoy nearer to home. Whether you travel near or far, there will always be an element of risk. Please keep a copy of your unique and very personal medical record at your fingertips. Dr. White provides an example (tool 1) for you to emulate on page 18.

Give the members of the health care team assembled to care for you — your better angels — their best chance to do their best for you. You will benefit and they and those near and dear to you will love you for it.

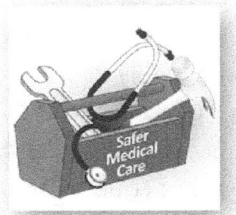

TOOL 1

My (Unique and Very) Personal Medical Record

Based upon my training and experience, I advocate that as your first order of business you review the gift example that follows immediately below: *My (Unique and Very) Personal Medical Record*. Once you have a basic understanding of the example, then emulate it by creating your own unique and very personal medical record. As you proceed, you may wish to contact me at drmikewhite@tmichaelwhitemd.com or safermedcare@gmail.com for clarifications or to request a formatted Microsoft Word example document so you may erase its example content and enter your own. I will be pleased to hear from you.

As you begin, a very important caveat: provided my training and my experience and consistent feedback from physicians and patients, I advocate a two page (maximum) document that approximates the following:

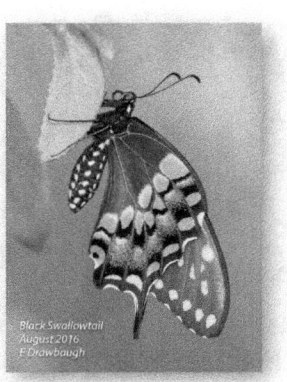

Black Swallowtail
August 2016
F.Drawbaugh

Tool 1: My (Unique and Very) Personal Medical Record — a gift example
Personal and Confidential

My Identification:

- Thomas Michael Example MD; DOB: ##/##/####
- Paradise Bay; 555-555-5555; mikeexamplemd@zmail.com
- Career: physician, educator, executive, talk show host; author
- My HealthCare Power of Attorney: Ms. Jacquelyn F Example (spouse); Paradise Bay; 555-555-5555

My Chief Complaint (my story — why I am here today):

For anticipated appointments, I will be prepared (in writing) to discuss the "O-P-Q-R2-S-T" of today's encounter: onset (when it started); place (what part of body); quality (what it feels like); related symptoms; radiation (where it travels to); severity (scale of 1-10); and triggers (what causes it, makes it worse or makes it better) — *after Dr. Orly Avitzur/Yale and others.*

My Allergies:

- Lifetime history of allergic rhinitis — **active**
- ACE inhibitors (for example, captopril) cause me to cough — **active**
- Respiratory depression with procedural sedation and analgesia — **active**
- No known allergies to medications
- No known allergy to latex

My Chronological Problem List:

Active:

- 1952 allergic rhinitis — active
- 1978 removal of multiple basal cell carcinomas — active
- 1978 actinic keratosis — active
- 1978 gastroesophogeal reflux disease (GERD) — active
- 1995 hypertension — active
- 1995 intolerance to ACE Inhibitors (cough) — active
- 1998 rosacea — active
- 2005 low HDL cholesterol — active
- 2011 pre-diabetes — active
- 2013 sleep apnea — active
- 2014 coronary artery disease — active
- 2014 left trochanteric bursitis; left sciatica (L5/S1); left cervical radiculopathy — active
- 2016 immunizations: Influenza (2016); Pneumovax (2015); Tdap; 2012; Zoster (2012); Hepatitis B (1995)
- 2016 cancer detection: gastroscopy (2000); colonoscopy (2010); PSA (2016)

Resolved:

- 1961 appendectomy — resolved
- 2003 cystoscopy and partial prostatectomy for benign prostatic hypertrophy — resolved
- 2005 left inguinal hernia repair — resolved
- 2006 hemorrhoid surgery — resolved

My Medication and Therapies List:

Allergic Rhinitis:

- Claritin (loratidine); 10mg; by mouth; once daily at bedtime
- Fluticasone nasal spray; 50 mcg; once daily (as necessary; rarely used)

- Azithromycin Z pack; 250 mg; by mouth; as directed for sinusitis (rarely used)
- Virtussin (guaifenesin/codeine phosphate) AC Syrup ; one teaspoon; by mouth; as directed for severe cough (rarely used)

Prompt: Remember Behavioral Health Conditions (for example, depression):
- *List medications and therapies*

Gastroesophageal Reflux Disease (GERD):
- Prilosec (omeprazole); 20 mg; by mouth; once daily at bedtime

Hyperlipidemia/Coronary Artery Disease:
- Lipitor (atorvastatin); 20mg; by mouth; once daily at bedtime
- Aspirin; 81mg; by mouth; once daily at bedtime

Hypertension:
- Cozaar (losartan); 100 mg; by mouth; once daily at bedtime

Prompt: Remember Ophthalmic Conditions (for example, glaucoma):
- *List medications and drops*

Prompt: Remember Pulmonary Conditions (for example, COPD):
- *List medications and Inhalers*

Rosacea:
- Metronidazole topical cream; 0.75%; apply to face daily

Sleep:
- CPAP; Nasal pillows (small); 7cm water; 3.5% humidity
- Ambien (zolpidem); 5 mg; by mouth; once daily at bedtime if necessary (rarely used)

Over-The-Counter medications (for example, vitamins):
- Tylenol (acetaminophen); 1000 mg; by mouth; every eight hours if necessary for fever or pain (rarely used)
- Advil (ibuprofen); 400-600 mg; by mouth; twice daily as necessary for activity related pain (used several times each week)

My Pertinent Family History

My paternal grandfather suffered with late life depression (87). My maternal grandfather died with senile dementia (74). My maternal grandmother died of renal cell carcinoma (85). My father died at 89. He struggled with hypertension, minor strokes and anxiety/depression. My mother is a breast cancer survivor and is alive and well (92). My siblings and children are alive and well.

My Personal Physicians:

- Cardiologist: Dr. Chester Paine/Paradise Bay/555-555-5555
- Dentist: Dr. Floss Daily/Paradise Bay/555-555-5555
- Dermatologist: Dr. U. V. Light/Paradise Bay/555-555-5555
- Gastroenterologist: Dr. Colin Reddy/Paradise Bay/555-555-5555
- General Surgeon: Dr. G. B. Stone/Paradise Bay/555-555-5555
- Interventional Cardiologist: Dr. Stent Thrombosis/Paradise Bay/555-555-5555
- Primary Care Physician: Dr. Wm. Osler Nodes/Paradise Bay/555-555-5555
- Orthopedist: Dr. Cairo Practer/Paradise Bay/555-555-5555
- Optometrist: Dr. Venus Blind/Paradise Bay/555-555-5555
- Radiologist: Dr. L. Azer Vision/Paradise Bay/555-555-5555
- My Personal Professional Patient Advocate (My P3A): Dr. Grace Wisdom/Paradise Bay/555-555-5555
- Pulmonary/Critical Care: Dr. Stephanie O. Scope /555-555-5555

My Significant HealthCare Attachments (available upon requests):

- 2015-01-09 cardiac cath report, baseline EKG and lab studies
- 2015-07-31 My (Unique and Very) Personal HealthCare Values/Wishes
- 2014-01-05 My HealthCare Advanced Directives

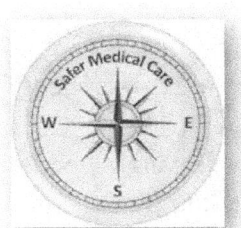

Safer Medical Care for You and Yours
www.tmichaelwhitemd.com; drmikewhite@tmichaelwhitemd.com
www.safermedcare.com; safermedcare@gmail.com

Dr. Stephen Hightower Comments

If you are like me, when I first came to an understanding of Dr. White's example — My (Unique and Very) Personal Medical Record — I had to take a deep breath, relax, and go, "wow, that is really a lot of data." It also reminded me of a recent trip to Glacier National Park in Montana. I was looking west over St. Mary's Lake and Goose Island, and after several moments just through my arms in the air and said, "OK this is perfect!" There is great value in appreciating perfect.

However, Dr. White has not infrequently reminded me that sometimes the biggest obstacle towards "good" is insistence upon perfection. Let me remind you that in 1969 we landed a man on the moon — the perfect Apollo 11. Astronaut Jim Lovell suggests NASA had half the PhDs on the planet working on this project. The numbering sequence in the Apollo series is a bit convoluted but please realize there were at least five Apollo designated missions prior to perfection. If NASA needs 6 trials before it can get to perfect, I am very happy to give myself some leeway in getting to perfect.

The important message is you must begin. As you approach perfect you will be forced to better understand your medical status, your medical conditions, your medications, your allergies and, very importantly, forced to identify and appoint your HealthCare Power of Attorney and her/his contact information. With each improvement, the better angels assembled to care for you will be increasingly positioned to provide you safe, effective compassionate care.

To get started, let me remind you that almost all doctors' offices are now computerized. At my office we use EPIC. This program assists you to get started by providing you what we call a snapshot which has on it your major medical problems, medications, and allergies. Ask your doctor for a similar printout and see how that document assists you move forward.

It is my experience that you will be proud of and find comfort in the document you create. It is my experience that you will then help your cherished love ones complete their own documents so they too may find peace and comfort in enabling safe, effective compassionate care.

Dr. White has placed contact information at the end of the above gift example. Should you require clarifications, he and his staff will be happy to assist you to quickly get you to good and, like NASA, moving towards perfect.

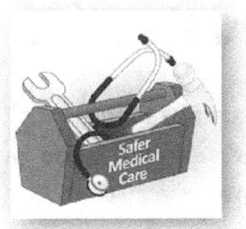

TOOL 2

My Chief Complaint
(my story — why I am here today)

Let us backtrack for a moment to the above gift example — *My (Unique and Very) Personal Medical Record* and consider the section: *My Chief Complaint (my story — why I am here today).*
With your *My (Unique and Very) Personal Medical Record* at your fingertips, through training and experience the better angels assembled to care for you will immediately understand the patient before them. At this point, it is critical that you be prepared to concisely and accurately answer their first question: "what brings you here today?" Through teaching/learning and practice, you must be able to efficiently convey (orally or even better, when circumstances allow, in writing) the "O-P-Q-R2-S-T" of today's encounter: onset (when it started); place (what part of body); quality (what it feels like); related symptoms; radiation (where it travels to); severity (scale of 1-10); and triggers (what causes it, makes it worse or makes it better). *Note: this pneumonic "O-P-Q-R2-S-T" is similar to one used by Yale's Dr. Orly Avitzur and others.*

What should this look like? Here is a reasonable hand-written facsimile — sure to put a relaxed smiley face on the busier-than-God better angels assembled to care for you:

My Chief Complaint (my story — why I am here today)

Thank you for seeing me today. As you can see by a quick review of My (Unique and Very) Personal Medical Record, I have basically been blessed with good health — a little of this and a little of that. However, starting about six weeks ago almost every time I walk up the hill to the 17th green, I get a sensation in my chest. It feels like a painful pressure. Sometimes it radiates into my neck and arm. At the same time, I get slightly short of breath and a little sweaty. On a scale of 1 to 10, it is never more than a four. As soon as I sit and rest, it passes. I happened to mention this to a nurse friend who is a bit of a patient advocate for me and she said I should check in with you immediately.

I anticipate that you readily see care efficiently and effectively moving in the right direction. As the story goes, the patient was sent directly for a cardiac catheterization. After review, blood pressure, lipid and lifestyle interventions were implemented. Her/his golf game has not improved.

Despite my self-imposed pressure to realize a concise brochure, I am compelled to demonstrate what the answer to the question, "What brings you here today?" must not look like. Please (please) avoid an inefficient, unhelpful, windy, uninterruptable response such as this:

"Doc, I should be playing golf. As I am sure you read in the paper, I finished sixth in the senior club championship. I would have won but I threw my putter in the lake and had to putt the last seven holes with my five-wood.

You know, you should have some golf magazines in the waiting room. By the way, are you aware that your magazines are a little on the moldy-oldie side? They go back to President Bush — President H. W. Bush.

Anyway, I am here because my wife, Mary, is a nervous Nellie. She's visiting her sick sister in Charleston or she would be here today chatting you up. Charleston is just too hot and muggy for me at this time of the year. But, I do like the food. Her sister had her gall bladder out and needs some help for a few days.

My wife made this appointment for me. She thinks I need a check-up. She thinks my little yellow pills need adjusting. She's the one who should be here — not as young as she used to be.

So Doc, do your thing and get me out of here for my 4 p.m. tee time. The boys are playing the back nine at the municipal course and I would hate to miss out. As you know, they have the best burgers in town. Since I am "baching it" tonight, if I survive this visit and the 17th hole, I might just have two..."

Quoting the poet, "Heaven help us all."

Dr. Stephen Hightower Comments

I learn so much from you. You tell me about your talents, your jobs, your visions of a good life and your hopes for your children, your country, and this world. These are important for us to share as it helps me to see you in the context of your world and helps me understand how you may envision me as a part of that experience.

But today I must focus with you on a symptom, or a specific concern. Something that is serious enough in your mind for you to take the time to come and see me. To do my best job, I need exacting information that allows me to pinpoint a single or perhaps several physical or mental processes that could be responsible for what you feel. Dr. White has introduced to you a very useful pneumonic — O-P-Q-R2-S-T — which most physicians employ when trying to better understand all the nuances of a symptom or problem. With our pneumonic driven information we begin to mentally construct the disease options which might be creating your disturbed feelings. From there, tests to narrow our possible explanations are ordered and evaluated to pinpoint the root cause of the ailment.

Several benefits are provided by your thoughtfully rehearsed My Chief Complaint (my story — why I am here today). First, you have already thought through these areas thus allowing more time at the visit for even more in-depth inquiry. Second and equally valuable, we can narrow the possible causes more efficiently and thus save you the cost of ordering unnecessary testing and return visits. With so many of us now having high deductible health plans, I would prefer to find and treat the diagnosis/cause with the least expenditure of hard earned assets.

With you informed, involved and responsible, we enter a collaborative effort that will help us get you diagnosed and on the road to wellness faster.

Once we have efficiently solved your problem or identified the path and testing needed to identify its source, let's make sure we use the time your preparations have provided me to discuss those other critical topics you have: like your most recent trip to Indonesia to photograph butterflies; your grand-daughters first piano recital; how you use a mule to keep a bull cow from walking through fences; and, of course, how to improve the soil for growing goji berries.

I really do learn so much from you.

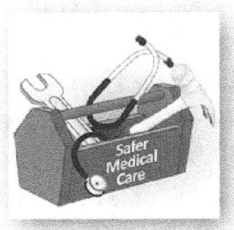

TOOL 3

My (Unique and Very) Personal HealthCare Values/Wishes

With your unique and very personal organized and accurate medical record in order (tool 1), tool 3 has you get in touch with your unique and very personal healthcare values and then construct a document that reflects your unique and very personal wishes.

It is natural for individuals to have trouble getting started on this emotionally charged document. However, it is my experience that, when working with the gift example that follows, the process efficiently moves forward. As you proceed, you will find that you must address some feelings and some technicalities that you have yet to address — for example, who do you desire to be your HealthCare Power(s) of Attorney? Although at first a bit daunting, it is my experience that you will find peace and well-being after successfully completing this document. Note: once completed, it is vital to share the document and clarify your exact meanings with your carefully selected HealthCare Power(s) of Attorney.

Now, I advocate you review the gift example: *My (Unique and Very) Personal HealthCare Values/Wishes* that immediately follows and then emulate it by creating your own unique and very personal document. As mentioned before, as you proceed, you may wish to contact me at drmikewhite@tmichaelwhitemd.com or safermedcare@gmail.com for clarifications or to request a formatted Microsoft Word example document so you may erase its example content and enter your own. I will be pleased to hear from you.

An important caveat: this document will only come to the attention of your assembled healthcare team in complex times. Unlike your concise two page *My (Unique and Very) Personal Medical Record*, you may and are encouraged to create an expansive narrative. In this regard, more is more.

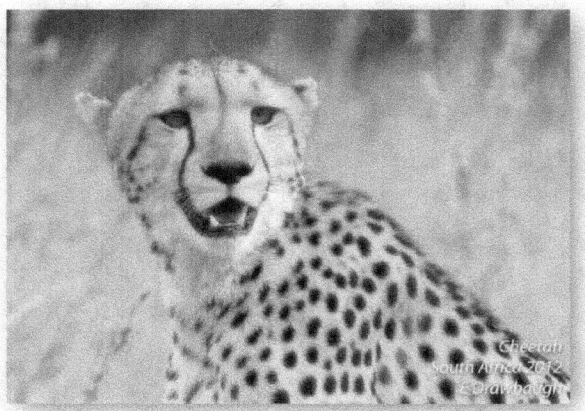

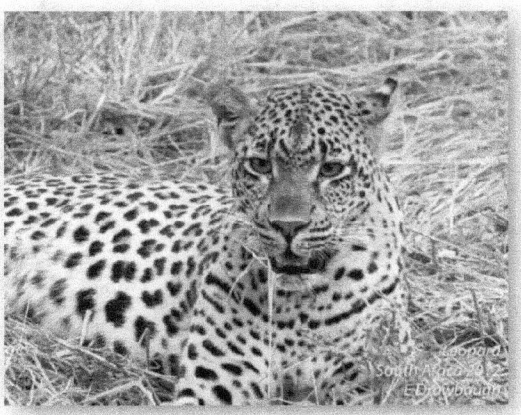

Tool 3: My (Unique and Very) Personal HealthCare Values/Wishes — a gift example
Personal and Confidential

My Identification

- T (Thomas) Michael Example MD; DOB: ##/##/####
- Paradise Bay; 555-555-5555; <u>mikeexamplemd@zmail.com</u>
- Career: physician, educator, executive, talk show host; author
- My HealthCare Power of Attorneys: Ms. Jacquelyn F Example (spouse); Paradise Bay; 555-555-5555; Mr. Colin Michael Example (son); Paradise Bay; 555-555-5555

My (Unique and Very) Personal HealthCare Values/Wishes

Two very special individuals in my life have been thoughtfully chosen and have and agreed to be appointed my HealthCare Power of Attorney. I thank them for that. As important:

- They have given me permission to share my considered thoughts about my unique and very personal wishes for the end of my life with them and
- They have spoken with me to clarify the meaning of my wishes with me.

They are prepared to speak for me should I lose the capacity to speak for myself as they understand…

Provided the wonderful meticulous compassionate care that has been afforded to me over the years, at this time I enjoy good health and I very much enjoy my life.

If I were to unexpectedly become seriously ill and there were to be a reasonable chance for my recovery, I wish to receive all indicated treatment to advance my recovery.

At the same time:

- *I comfortably recognize death as a part of life.*
- *If a meaningful recovery were to be unlikely, I would prefer a dignified death.*
- *For emphasis and clarification, I would place no value in preserving my life if heart, lungs and kidneys function but my wits, as I now know and enjoy them, have departed.*
- *For emphasis and clarification, very specifically, if two qualified physicians using an approved protocol determine that I am brain dead or in a persistent vegetative state, please recognize that I have died and proceed accordingly. In such circumstances, I place no value in preserving my life and desire interventions to maintain my life (for example, feeding tubes, antibiotics, transfusions, ventilators, dialysis, etc.) not be implemented or, if already implemented, be withdrawn.*
- *For further clarification, I would recognize a prolonged existence in such a state as a major terminal indignity to a life well lived — an indignity to be avoided.*
- *At the same time, should I desire "not to be resuscitated", I request that this not be interpreted as "not to be cared for." I request, in every circumstance (recovery or terminal), that my healthcare team continuously attend to my dignity and ensure my comfort. Confidence that my dignity and comfort will be addressed is very important and reassuring to me.*

Background Information

A. **My Unique (and Very) Personal Medical Record**

   Please refer to an attached separate document — *My Unique (and Very) Personal Medical Record* which provides you with an efficient, organized and accurate understanding of my past and current medical care. Thank you.

B. **Purpose**

   The purpose of this document — *My (Unique and Very) Personal HealthCare Values/Wishes* — is to efficiently and effectively convey in complex circumstances (for example, when I have lost the capacity to speak for myself):

   - The very unique person I am and
   - My unique and very personal healthcare values

to the fine, dedicated and caring healthcare team assigned to my care and to my HealthCare Power(s) of Attorney designated in my attached Healthcare Advanced Directive. I anticipate that this will ensure that care is provided in accordance with my values and wishes. This is very important and comforting to me.

I have constructed this document with great care. It reflects in-depth conversation with my family, my HealthCare Power of Attorney and with significant others in my life. In constructing this document, it has been my intent to:

- Advance the professional vitality of the fine dedicated and caring healthcare team caring for me by saving them precious time and energy through removing ambivalence and uncertainty about my values and wishes,
- Position myself to enable and receive safer, timely, efficient, effective and equitable (fair/just) patient-centered medical care by providing organized and accurate information,
- Do my involved, informed and responsible part to advance the HealthCare Value that my healthcare team provides to me (for me, HealthCare Value *equates* to compassionate medical care; quality outcomes; patient and staff safety; customer (patient, family and community) satisfaction; patient advocacy; and professional (medical, nursing, professional and support staffs') vitality *balanced by* resource utilization/cost and
- Ensure that my very personal healthcare values and wishes are understood (by me, my family, my healthcare powers of attorney and my healthcare team) and honored.

C. **My Personal Information — My Social History**

It is important to me that the better angels caring for me in complex circumstances appreciate the unique and very special (to some) person I am — to that end, I have had the honor and privilege to be a physician (general internist). My responsibilities have included private practice, residency program direction, graduate medical education (vice president value and education) and hospital administration (vice president medical affairs/chief medical officer). I have surveyed for The Joint Commission and the Accreditation Council for Graduate Medical Education. At this time, I am a HealthCare Value (quality, safety, experience, advocacy and vitality balanced by cost) author and consultant. I am on a mission to advance each individual's safer medical care by assisting her/him to be an informed, involved and responsible patient.

I grew up as a blue collar kid in Schenectady, New York. Along the way, I have been blessed to be influenced and nurtured by Union College, Albany Medical College, New York Medical College, Yale University, the University of Connecticut, the University of Arizona, Temple University, Michigan State University and the University of Pittsburgh. I live with my wife, Jacquelyn F Example RN BSN (555-555-5555). We have four successful children of whom we are very proud. They live with their families in Santa Barbara (Benjamin), Louisville (Jessica), Arlington (Catherine) and Washington DC (Colin). In my spare time I enjoy studying medicine, writing, negotiating the New York Times, competitive golf, competitive poker, music, cinema, boating (Lake George) and thoroughbred racing (Saratoga).

D. **Expectations**

Through the creation and maintenance of this document, I have striven to provide the members of my healthcare team and my healthcare power(s) of attorney with the necessary and accurate information required to address my care in a compassionate, efficient and effective manner. Should additional information or complex decision making (for example, informed consent) be required, I anticipate you will approach me.

In the circumstance where I lack the capacity to communicate, I anticipate my healthcare team will address concerns with my healthcare power(s) of attorney (identified in my attached Healthcare Advanced Directive) who are well informed of my values and wishes.

I expect that my personal values will be respected and my wishes will be honored. I expect that my attending physician will write orders that are compatible with my values and that my healthcare team will follow those orders.

E. Informed Consent

I anticipate that my healthcare team and my healthcare institution will:

- Procure informed consent prior to the implementation of any complex procedure or treatment;
- As part of informed consent, assist with an informed understanding of complex financial implications of my care (for example, the hospital accepts my insurance but the physicians providing care do not);
- Whenever informed consent is required, ask me and
- If the circumstance is such that I have lost the capacity to speak for myself, then, obtain informed consent from my HealthCare Power(s) of Attorney identified in my attached Healthcare Advanced Directive. Through detailed dialogue with me, these individuals understand my very personal healthcare values and wishes; will respect them; and are entirely prepared to speak on my behalf with my interest at heart. Through detailed dialogue with me, they are prepared to work with my attending physician and complete my circumstance dependent end of life directives (for example, my Maryland Medical Orders for Life-Sustaining Treatment (MOLST) form) if I am unable to do so.

F. My Personal Professional Patient Advocate (My P3A):

Should I unexpectedly become severely ill, I anticipate that my healthcare process may become complex. Therefore, I anticipate that I or my HealthCare Power(s) of Attorney may engage, at our own expense, a *My Personal Professional Patient Advocate (My P3A)* who:

- Understands the complexity of the healthcare process,
- Will be adopted/deputized/appointed as a family member (and not as a member of my healthcare team),
- Will, upon my request or upon the request of my HealthCare Power(s) of Attorney, review my chart and participate in family meetings, etc.,
- Will assist me and and/or my HealthCare Power(s) of Attorney in understanding my care (i.e., act as interpreter for the purpose of making the complex simple) and
- Will assist with the respectful, efficient, effective and articulate communication of my personal healthcare values and wishes to my healthcare team.

Should a My P3A be engaged, please welcome this very carefully identified and selected adopted/deputized/appointed family member into my family and into my care.

(*Note for clarification: although my P3A's opinion may prove invaluable to my decision-making process, decisions will be made by me or, when necessary, by my HealthCare Power(s) of Attorney.*

G. Complexity

Through the process of creating this document — *My (Unique and Very) Personal HealthCare Values/Wishes* — I have striven to diminish (and I do not anticipate) the possibility of clinical, ethical or legal complexity. I fully expect that my personal healthcare values and wishes will be respected and honored. I fully expect that my attending physician will write orders that are compatible with my personal healthcare values and wishes and that my healthcare team will follow those orders.

Should legal or ethical complexity arise, I fully expect, request and insist the healthcare institution's ethics committee process:

- Review this document ,
- Speak with me or if I do not have the capacity to communicate, speak with my HealthCare Power(s) of Attorney,
- Upon my request or at the request of my HealthCare Power(s) of Attorney, include *My Personal Professional Patient Advocate (My P3A)* in discussions so *My P3A* is positioned to offer perspective, advice and counsel to my decision-making process and

- Resolve any ambiguity in favor of my personal healthcare values and wishes by sundown (i.e., within 24 hours).

H. Gratitude

I recognize that my healthcare team is comprised of our nation's "best and brightest." I recognize that through dedication, sacrifice and experience you have become "better angels" in my life.

I am most appreciative of and confident in your care. I thank you for being here for me today.

Attachment #1: 2014-01-03 My HealthCare Advance Directive

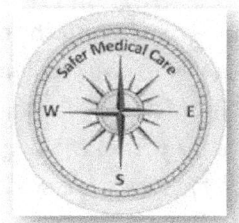

Safer Medical Care for You and Yours
www.tmichaelwhitemd.com; drmikewhite@tmicahelwhitemd.com
www.safermedcare.com; safermedcare@gmail.com

Dr. Stephen Hightower Comments

I have been watching you and learning of your values for a lifetime.

I heard of your values as young boy, listening to you talk of serving your country on an aircraft carrier in the Pacific at age 18. At that time, I was not sure what you meant when you said all of your friends did not get to come home. I observed your values as I went with you regularly to deliver the little knitted caps and shawls to the hospital for the newborns. Yet, I was surprised because I knew I had to get the cups off the shelf for you because of your severe hand arthritis. I felt your values when I was stopped at school to discuss my second grade son's class work, and you were there with several others trying to help him and the other children with their reading.

After my lifetime of observation, I am now ready to pay you back and to pay it forward. For you see, now your values have become my values. I want to example what you have taught me to others and I want to help you identify your thoughts that will allow us to care for you in the way you wish as time moves forward. To do that, reflections such as those above, about your own life experiences that honed your own set of values and influenced how you conducted your life will help. Dr. White has provided you examples of specific personal healthcare values; a way of describing your social history; expectations you might outline for your health care team; the concept of informed consent; and the value of a personal, professional, patient advocate. Read through these gifts and use them as ground work for you or your HealthCare Power of Attorney to deliver to your care team your statement of your unique self, the unique role you have had in this life and the unique way you want your team to care for you in the future.

As we chat, I am remembering wise childhood (second grade) advice that still works well today: "Do not cry because it is over, but smile that it happened." Dr. Seuss

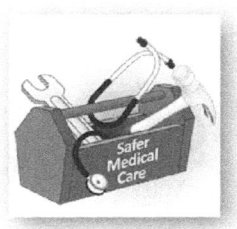

TOOL 4

My HealthCare Power of Attorney (and My Advanced Directives)

For reasons that are unclear to me, as soon as advanced directives are mentioned, we run for shelter and hunker down. Let me simplify it and make it less daunting:

- Create a will (a good idea);
- Consider who you want to be your legal power of attorney if/when circumstances dictate (a good idea);
- Identify and appoint your HealthCare Power of Attorney (a must do);
- Get in touch with your unique and personal healthcare values/wishes and commit them to writing (what an idea); and then
- Review your values/wishes with your HealthCare Power of Attorney (a must do).

After review, that was not so bad.

As you addressed your unique and very personal medical record and your unique and very personal healthcare values, you clarified in your own mind your HealthCare Power(s) of Attorney — the person(s) who will speak for you if you do not have the capacity to speak for yourself — so that is already done. So now, as the kids say, chat her/him up.

A couple of important caveats:

Your HealthCare Power of Attorney must both agree to accept the responsibility and agree to give you permission and time to discuss and clarify your wishes;

- Your legal advance directives appoint people to roles. Carefully avoid specific rigid actions to be taken in specific circumstances. When the time comes, those decisions will be made in the context of your circumstances by you or, when necessary, by your HealthCare Power of Attorney who, through on-going communications with you, will understand the decisions you would make/want to be made in any unanticipated unique and complex circumstance.
- For clarification, an important example: my own personal health care advanced directives document formally appoints my chosen HealthCare Power(s) of Attorney; but, in the section for living will it very specifically and consciously states: "living will intentionally omitted." If/when the time comes, my HealthCare Power of Attorney will refer to *My (Unique and Very Personal) HealthCare Values/Wishes*, remember our conversations and make specific decisions on my behalf in concert with my well-articulated and well understood wishes.

Dr. Stephen Hightower Comments

I see you are admiring my picture of Lou Gehrig. I have had that picture of Mr. Gehrig giving his farewell speech at Yankee Stadium in one of my exam rooms for over 20 years. No, I'm not really a Yankee's fan. I'm just a Lou Gehrig fan.

Why? Well here is a young man at the age of 35 who is at the top of his game. He is recognized by all of his peers and the public as one of the true stars of his profession for both his athletic prowess and his gentlemanly values. Then after 14 years of exceptional play, he begins to develop weakness and his play is significantly affected. He is eventually diagnosed with amyotrophic lateral sclerosis, a degenerative neurologic disease, which now bears his name — Lou Gehrig's disease.

Amyotrophic lateral sclerosis is universally fatal. Although today we can control many of the symptoms with technology and thus prolong life, there is no cure. As in Mr. Gehrig's day, it is simply a death sentence.

On July the 4th 1939 he gave his farewell address to 62,000 fans at Yankee Stadium saying, "Today I consider myself the luckiest man on the face of this earth." That statement, in that setting, demonstrates his ability to control his mind and thus control his world. Mr. Gehrig's personal values in his life were not lost but were accentuated and were available to him as he stayed in control of how his life would progress from that point forward.

And that is what we are concerned about today. I want you to be in control of what happens to you as your life moves forward. Mr. Gehrig had some time to prepare himself and his family, not everyone gets that chance. An advanced directive and the appointment of your very thoughtfully personally selected HealthCare Power of Attorney allows you to provide your doctors with the understanding of what you want us to do for you so you remain in control. Were you aware that on national surveys over 80% of people hope to die at home but only 20-30% actually do? The resources to allow a dignified death at home are better now than ever before. However the complexity of balancing treatments, be they lifesaving or life prolonging, with your very personal values and desires needs your input or that of your HealthCare Power of Attorney with whom you have discussed your wishes.

Most doctors have forms for Advanced Directives in the office. States vary on the need for a notary or the legal provisions for identifying someone as your HealthCare Power of Attorney. This is a very important issue. Remember Mr. Gehrig, by example, teaches us control. Control your world and fill out that Advanced Directive and converse regularly with your HealthCare Power of Attorney. Do not blindly trust the medical system will do what is best. We can only do our best when you give us guidance on how to approach challenging issues from your very unique perspective.

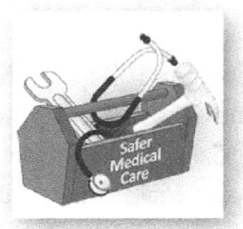

My Personal Professional Patient Advocate (My P3A)

As you considered Tool 3: *My (Unique and Very) Personal HealthCare Values/Wishes*, you encountered the concept of *My Personal Professional Patient Advocate (My P3A)*. I apologize for this seemingly out of sequence frasm. Let's clear that up. Thorough experience, I have come to understand:

- Non-legal people benefit from legal counsel when confronted with complex legal circumstances (for example, a court appearance). Lawyers are frequently engaged;
- Non-financial people benefit from financial counsel when confronted with complex financial circumstances (for example, an IRS audit). Accountants are frequently engaged.
- In the same vein, non-medical people benefit from a medical advocate when confronted with complex medical circumstances (for example, admission to the hospital); however, medical advocates are infrequently engaged;
- My family and friends have the benefit of a physician advocate (me) to understand and translate complex medical circumstances. They often engage me to do so; but
- Many individuals (and their HealthCare Power(s) of Attorney) are not medically sophisticated and would benefit from a medical advocate. For example, although my HealthCare Power of Attorney is an experienced favorite nurse (my spouse), I have a trusted medically sophisticated advocate (a senior clinician and physician executive) in the wings who may be engaged to run interference if/when I or my HealthCare Power of Attorney believe it necessary.

Therefore, I advocate that each of us identify a *My Personal Professional Patient Advocate (My P3A)* who can be consulted if and when complex circumstances dictate. The language from tool 3, the gift example *My (Unique and Very) Personal HealthCare Values/Wishes*, clarifies how my personal *My P3A* will function and is repeated here:

My Personal Professional Patient Advocate (My P3A)

Should I unexpectedly become severely ill, I anticipate that my healthcare process may become complex. Therefore, I anticipate that I or my HealthCare Power(s) of Attorney may engage, at our own expense, a *My Personal Professional Patient Advocate (My P3A)* who:

- Understands the complexity of the healthcare process,
- Will be adopted/deputized/appointed as a family member (and not as a member of my healthcare team),
- Will, upon my request or upon the request of my HealthCare Power(s) of Attorney, review my chart and participate in family meetings, etc.,
- Will assist me and and/or my HealthCare Power(s) of Attorney in understanding my care (i.e., act as interpreter for the purpose of making the complex simple), and
- Will assist with the respectful, efficient, effective and articulate communication of my personal healthcare values and wishes to my healthcare team.

Should a My P3A be engaged, please welcome this very carefully identified and selected adopted/deputized/appointed family member into my family and into my care.

(Note for clarification: although my P3A's opinion may prove invaluable to my decision-making process, decisions will be made by me or, when necessary, by my HealthCare Power(s) of Attorney).

Dr. Stephen Hightower Comments

A "hypothetical" composite true story — I address them every day — to illustrate why we all need a Personal Professional Patient Advocate.

John and Mary: I was happy to see your father as you requested, in order to give you some insights on his situation. Thank you for a copy of your father's Unique and Personal Medical Record and Healthcare Values/Wishes. Even though I am privileged at the hospital where he was admitted, without permission it is a HIPPA violation for me to examine his records, so the information you provided helped me when talking to your dad's attending surgeon and the hospitalist caring for him today.

Until four months ago it sounds as if your father was the Mr. Active at his Adult Living community. His only medical problem was a history of prostate cancer treated with radiation therapy back in 2006. Then he began a slow progressive loss of 40 pounds and a marked decrease in muscle strength. He had multiple procedures with CT scans, scopes, and muscle tests, without an obvious cause.

Four days ago he became disoriented and he was hospitalized with findings of an elevated blood calcium level and an enlarged bladder. Fluids helped get the calcium down, and a catheter was placed in his bladder which revealed blood. An ultrasound of his kidneys showed that they were obstructed and swollen. The urologist placed a scope in the bladder and saw a bleeding prostate and a very distorted bladder. He could not put in drains to help the kidneys. The next day they placed an external tube into each kidney through his back. He currently continues to bleed from the prostate/bladder, his blood count is very low and he requires transfusions. There is concern that the elevated calcium is due to a tumor making a unique protein that causes the calcium to go up. When I saw him today he still smiled and was very kind and pleasant, but he did not recognize me though we have spoken several times in the past.

So where are we? Your wonderful father likely has an undiagnosed tumor; he has severe blood loss anemia from a hemorrhaging prostate that has already been radiated, he has a very abnormal bladder probably from the radiation of the prostate; and he has kidneys that cannot drain normally. He is asking for your guidance on how he should proceed. We know transfusions will treat his anemia. His specialists state his hemorrhaging prostate and bladder must be removed and an external pouch must be created to drain his kidneys — arduous surgeries for even a healthy patient. Thereafter, he will still need to address the yet to be diagnosed tumor.

So what do you do: choices almost always include treatment, palliative care, or hospice? How do you decide? You talk with the family and provide everyone the same knowledge on the situation. You listen. You discuss the situation with your dad and read his healthcare values. You listen.

You have a large family and it is possible there will not be complete unanimity in what you should do. Do not fear that. He has very thoughtfully and specifically chosen and entrusted you to make decisions on his behalf.

Should your father lose the capacity to make his own decisions that responsibility will fall to you. Being blessed with what your father has instructed you to do in the past and what he has so thoughtfully written, feel absolutely confident that you will make the right decision with the clear data he has provided to you.

Go forward without fear or regret. Go forward only with the peace of mind that he is grateful for and has tremendous peace of mind for your ministrations.

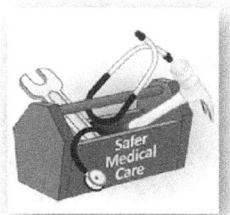

My Safer Medical Care Emergency Alert System

This is all about me. I am famously and accurately accused of being the guy with both suspenders and belt and both raincoat and umbrella — guilty as charged. Relevant to this discussion, I worry that with my medical record, my healthcare values and my HealthCare Power of Attorney all in order, I, without the capacity to speak for myself (for example, after a highway crash), will be brought to a strange emergency room with no information. Therefore, when traveling I have a two-sided business card in my shirt pocket and in my wallet that approximates:

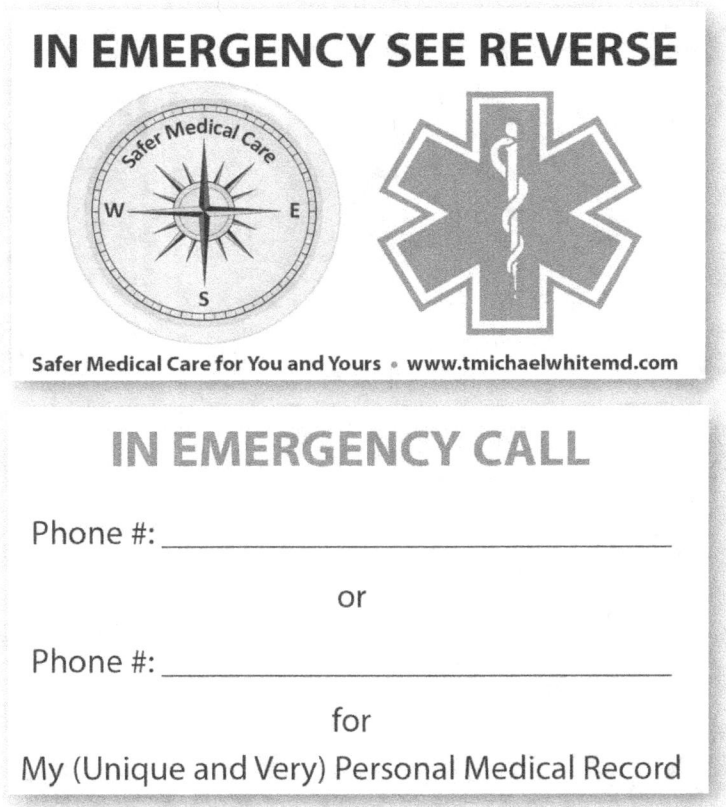

I travel frequently and always have the above business card in my shirt pocket and wallet. This approach:

- Works well in my shirt pocket and wallet;
- Can be readily updated;
- Can be copied from this brochure (please see last pages);
- Can be posted in on my refrigerator, in my hospital room; etc.; and
- Provides me with a sense of security that the right people will be involved if/when circumstances dictate.

For myself, I have chosen to have the mobile numbers for my HealthCare Powers of Attorney listed on my cards. Through planning they have ready access to *My (Unique and Very) Personal Medical Record*. Through clear communications, they understand my (unique and very) personal healthcare values and wishes. They are prepared to advance and honor my wishes if/when I am unable to do so. With this in place, whether I am on the road or at home, these business cards have come to provide me with tremendous peace of mind.

Dr. Stephen Hightower Comments

You and I have done significant work to prepare ourselves in case of an unforeseen emergency or accident. Now it is important to make sure our work gets into the hands of the people (the better angels) assembled to care for us. Multiple options exist.

I personally have a folded copy of Tool 1 — My (Unique and Very) Personal Medical Record — in my billfold. It is prominently labeled, "for Emergency Medical Personnel". It will work if someone checks my billfold. With the power of information — my medications, my allergies and the name and number of my HealthCare Power of Attorney — I am confident my care will move in the right direction.

Dr. Whites' wallet card suggestion is easily accomplishable and useful. You can make several copies and have them on your person, in your car, briefcase, purse, on your refrigerator door, etc. This ensures your treating better angels will have quick access to the information they need to treat you correctly and safely.

A third option is to be creative. Consider making up your own personal card. On it you can put, in a very brief way, something unique about you. Of course the information about who to call for your (Unique and Very) Personal Medical Record goes on the back. For instance, the title MD does inform people of my profession. However, few would know that I am an avid bicyclist who loves to ride in the US National Parks with my "To Boldly Go" Star Trek jersey on. It is ok to boldly shout out yourself — with the colors, designs, insignias, phrases and dreams on one side, and the number for your personal HealthCare Power(s) of Attorney on the back.

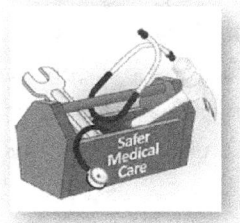

Towards a Well-Lived Life — A Dozen Practical Recommendations (Dr. White)

Without apology, I am on a mission to position you and yours for safe, effective compassionate care. To the best of my ability, I have shown you how to do it. Now I have to sell it to you. I have to address your very reasonable and very human question: "what's in it for me and mine?"

I became a complete physician when I too had to walk the walk of a patient. That experience demonstrated to me that I (the patient) had to do my part by preparing so the better angels assembled to care for me could effectively and compassionately practice their masterful craft on my behalf. The six tools I have crafted have been presented to you. I encourage you to follow my lead.

My career as a clinician, my experiences as a patient and family member and the process of writing this primer have encouraged me to step back and ask and attempt to answer a broader question — what should I be doing each day to advance a well-lived life? I have come up with a list of 12 recommended actions. I put them forward for your consideration. Importantly, in so doing, Dr. Hightower has the opportunity to comment. For my own edification (and yours), I very much look forward to his reactions and insights:

1. Be actively involved in, informed about and responsible for your healthcare;
2. Identify your (very thoughtfully selected) HealthCare Power(s) of Attorney;
3. Compose and keep your organized and accurate *My (Unique and Very) Personal Medical Record* at your fingertips;
4. As you address #3 understand and minimize your medications — less will almost always prove to be more;
5. Get in touch with your *My (Unique and Very) Personal Healthcare Values/Wishes* and commit them to writing;
6. Once composed, share #3, *My (Unique and Very) Personal Medical Record* and #5, *My (Unique and Very) Personal Healthcare Values/Wishes* with your HealthCare Power(s) of Attorney;
7. Become adept at efficiently conveying (for example, consciously script) your *My Chief Complaint (my story — why I am here today)* whenever presenting for complex care;
8. Engage daily in physical gymnastics — stretch comprehensively, gently pump some iron and moderately aerobically exercise;
9. Engage daily in mental gymnastics — keep abreast of local, national and world news (while at the same time transferring responsibility for the world's universal problems to the fine, capable younger generations that follow); write a journal; send thoughtful emails to and have substantive conversations with family and friends; and challenge, like Poirot, your "little gray cells" with math, crossword, card games and a murder mystery or two;
10. Eat and drink in moderation (for example, a Mediterranean diet) and maintain a reasonable weight;

11. Make sleep at night a priority and unashamedly expertly nap in the day; and

12. Be transformed by the continuous renewal of your mind. Consciously plan and enjoy cinema, literature, music, sporting events, theater, travel and spiritualties that suit you.

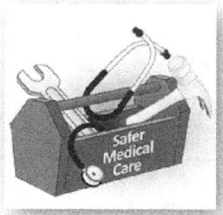

Towards a Well-Lived Life — Ten Philosophical Thoughts (Dr. Hightower)

r. White has struck a chord with his practical thoughts. Let me wax philosophically (surely my own book someday). Here is an abridged version...

Life is composed of physical activities and the thoughts which control those activities. Please consider incorporating the following ten thought activities so your mind helps you to always remain in control, regardless of what the physical world may present.

1. ***Control your World by Controlling Your Mind:*** *controlling your mind helps to eliminate the self-imposed fear or guilt we create in our lives. We can stop reacting to the random events in our world and control our thoughts. Then, with contemplation, we allow ourselves to identify the course we need to take based on who we are. Consider "Courage Under Fire" by James Bond Stockdale — a pamphlet of enduring value.*

2. ***Make One Thing in Life as Important as You:*** *when you do, you insert purpose in your life. Purpose ensures a meaningful existence.*

3. ***Challenge Yourself by Making and Reaching Goals:*** *small goals consistently reached provide the confidence and swagger that allow us to push out further. Because you control your mind, you deal with setbacks. Your purpose gives you the incentive to reach your goals.*

4. ***Embrace Change:*** *With 7 billion people on the planet, the world does not remain static. However, the world is not for us to control. We can control our mind, maintain our personal purpose, reach our goals and embrace change.*

5. ***Your Perception is Your Reality:*** *many years of life are not required to be successful, only your perception of those years is important. Hang a picture of Lou Gehrig and absorb his journey and his perceptions. Then go about taking each new day as a gift. Unlike yesterday and today, tomorrow will never be guaranteed. Feel positive about every moment you have had.*

6. ***Seek Out Inspiration:*** *we need a recurrent dose of inspiration to help break the tedium of performing our day to day responsibilities. Inspiration may be philosophical, physical, intellectual, or spiritual. It may come to you from nature, books, movies, speakers, artists, musicians, friends, or classes. Take the time to listen, absorb, feel, experience, touch, and think. This will help to ingrain in you the will to regularly interact with that which inspires you.*

7. ***Inspire Others:*** *my daily goal is to inspire others to be healthy and safe. It is a challenge. You will be inspiring to children, colleagues, friends, spouses and neighbors, if you simply live the 10 items in this list. Think about a personal plan to inspire those closest to you. Walk your talk. Use your actions and brief examples as often as words to inspire and encourage. Recognize, enjoy and replicate each success.*

8. **Cultivate a Poor Short Term Memory**: many of my patients have had medical challenges in which we encourage a change in life-style. Sometimes attempts at change fail. Your reaction should be to constantly adjust your approach based on the failed attempt, to set another goal and to push forward with encouragement. This is called resilience. We all fall short at times. As a strategic path to happiness, control your mind, feel your purpose, push towards your goals, recognize and embrace the obstacles, remember what inspired you and quickly forget failed attempts.

9. **It is All about Culture:** who you are and what you are is often very dependent on where you are physically. The culture of that space affects you tremendously as a person. Everything we have talked about previously is affected by the environment you are in and the outlook of the people around you. Choose a positive, growing, embracing and inspiring culture that facilitates our personal success. Then inspire others by sharing the culture that energizes and nourishes you.

10. **Consistency is King:** what have we ever done well that was not carefully prepared and consistently practiced? Consistent effort is required to maintain our mind in control. Consistent effort is required to prevent spontaneous emotions or outside events from ruling us. Consistently reinforce your commitments — your purpose. Consistently set forth and reach goals. Consistently appreciate and learn new things and embrace positive change. Consistently appreciate each day and relish its unique ups and downs. Consistently find inspiration. Consistently act in ways to inspire those who are privileged to encounter you daily. Consistently disarm failure and, with resilience, find a new, better path. Consistently seek out the people and growing, embracing and inspiring culture that facilitates your personal success to which you aspire.

Most importantly, consistently feel your active control of your world and dynamically control the quality of your life.

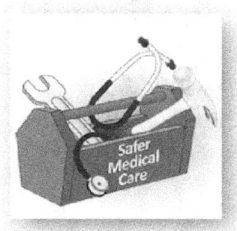

Another Charismatic Story:
Script to the Rescue

My first book used all too real powerful fictions to demonstrate why having your organized and *My (Unique and Very) Personal Medical Record* at your fingertips and why being able to articulate your *My Chief Complaint (my story — why I am here today)* must become an imperative for you. In a conscious effort to be concise, the stories have largely been eliminated — save for this one.

———⚭———

Before the abrupt onset of her incapacitating illness at age 60, she was, just like you and me, bullet-proof and invincible:

- She will never have an unanticipated illness and
- If she ever has an unanticipated illness, she and her spouse will merely explain, "until today I have been in the best of health, when…"

Then she had one of those elective same day surgeries women consider part of life. As the story goes, the surgery was unexpectedly prolonged. Almost immediately, she had some devastating neurological symptoms which included pain, weakness and incoordination. Her condition left her unable to concentrate or work. Eating became an exhausting chore and, thin to start, she lost significant weight.

Her superb small-town physicians were perplexed — flummoxed really. She and her spouse traveled several uncomfortable hours at significant expense to the university to see a neurological specialist who saw her for what seemed only several minutes; told her, with little explanation, she had a serious neurological condition; and pre-scribed a potent oral medication. No comprehensive testing, rehabilitation or follow-up was arranged. The first dose of the new prescription made her violently ill and she had no one to turn to. She and her husband found themselves doubly devastated, first by illness and now by a perceived lack of communication and compassionate care.

Complicating her situation, she was not native born and had some difficulty expressing herself in English (especially when emotional); her illness had left her quite emotional; and her brilliant, gentleman husband was by nature politely laconic. Recognizing they needed assistance in interfacing with their healthcare better angels, they identified a logical senior physician in their lives and adopted/deputized/assigned her as the patient's *My Personal Professional Patient Advocate (My P3A)*. Over the phone, the *My P3A* listened patiently and well and sent them a draft of the patient's own *My (Unique and Very) Personal Medical Record*. It was understood that a key to success was to have the patient's *My Chief Complaint (my story — why I am here today)* crisp and concisely in order. In preparation for a consultation with a carefully selected second neurologist, she and her *My P3A* constructed her story and committed it to writing for hand delivery to her super-specialist.

My Chief Complaint (my story — why I am here today)

I have enjoyed good health. Six months ago, I underwent same day, laparoscopic gynecological surgery. I was to receive twilight anesthesia but the procedure was more difficult and took much longer than expected. I suspect I may have been converted to general anesthesia.

Since that time (starting immediately thereafter) I have had significant difficulty with concentration (multitasking — my specialty — is now very difficult for me), coordination, fatigue, weakness, numbness and pain (8 0n a scale of 1-10) in my arms, hips and legs and an inability to sleep (because of significant discomfort). Since that time, I have been unable to work. Of late, my symptoms are the worst from my waist down. My handwriting has deteriorated and is often illegible. I have lost my appetite; I am too fatigued to eat and have lost 30 pounds. My fatigue, weakness and discomfort become more severe as the day progresses.

My personal physician diagnosed anxiety and prescribed Lorazepam (which numbed me) and Lexapro (which I could not take — muscle stiffness). In December, I saw a neurologist (MRI of head "normal") who after a very brief encounter diagnosed "a movement disorder" and prescribed Sinemet (which I could not take — muscle stiffness). An internist has recently prescribed Gabapentin which has provided some relief of my symptoms. He did not offer a diagnosis. He requests the opinion of a second neurologist.

The following transpired:

- Her better angel neurological consultant, aided by her concise My Chief Complaint (my story — why I am here today) was immediately positioned to think about (diagnose and treat) her.
- Based upon her history and a thorough neurological exam, a very rare acute movement disorder (possibly related to complications of anesthesia) was diagnosed and explained.
- A medication was prescribed. Indications and potential side effects were described in detail. The patient tolerated the medication. Her symptoms significantly abated.
- Very specialized testing, physical medicine and rehabilitation consultation (in her community) and timely follow-up with the neurological specialist were arranged.
- From the moment they met with the second neurologist, the patient and family immediately sensed movement from frightening powerless hopelessness to informed, interested compassionate comprehensive care — not a cure, but a guided journey well begun.

For me, this journey pulls my message together. It is our business to be involved in, informed about and responsible for our healthcare. The best way for us to accomplish this is for each of us to:

- Have our organized and accurate medical record at out fingertips;
- Be prepared to concisely state our concerns and
- Engage an advocate to assist with complexity

so our better angels are positioned to provide safe, effective compassionate care.

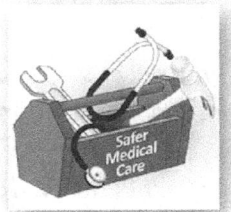

A Patient Speaks —
In Control, Safer and Relieved

wish to write in support of Dr. White's enthusiastic advocacy for each of us to be involved in, informed about and responsible for our healthcare. The best way to accomplish this is to share my own true story with you.

Back in the last millennium, when I was in my mid-50's, I had just one doctor, a general practitioner whom I had visited regularly for more than a decade. He may not have known everything about medicine, but he knew a lot about me. If a medical problem surfaced that was above his pay grade, he took the time to research it, sometimes consulting a specialist and then took more time to explain the situation to me and what we could do about it.

So when routine blood tests revealed that something was preventing my blood from clotting, we talked some more, he ordered additional tests that ruled out the more sinister possibilities and we settled into a watch and wait mode. He retired a few years later and I moved into the new millennium and the age of modern healthcare.

My new primary care physician was caring and courteous, but he really didn't have the time to get to know me or to wade through the foot-thick medical record I had deposited at the front desk. When my clotting problem got worse, my third new PCP ordered more tests and consulted more specialists. My physicians still hadn't found the cause of my symptoms, but the problem hadn't yet reached a critical stage, so watch and wait was still the path to follow. When one of the team recommended that I undergo a necessary simple outpatient surgical procedure, the consensus was, "Go ahead. It shouldn't be a problem."

The procedure was simple, but it took five hospitalizations at two different hospitals to stop the uncontrolled bleeding that followed. By the time I was discharged, I had a half-dozen specialists who examined and tested me regularly, prescribed remedies as needed and sounded the alarm if they detected a potential health threat.

You'd think that all this attention would be reassuring. In a way it was, but I also felt like the elephant in the "Blind Men and the Elephant" fable. Regularly one or more of the doctors wouldn't get the message about a new symptom, test result, or prescription change. Normally there was time to ultimately get everyone on the same page, but I knew that if my bleeding problem got critical, I might be in for another marathon hospital tour or worse.

Fortunately, while my wife was editing his first book, Dr. White *agreed to be My Personal Professional Patient Advocate (My P3A)*. He didn't call it that. He merely said, "Let me listen to your complex story and show you how to organize it so you are positioned to enable and receive safer medical care." With his help, I developed my own *My (Unique and Very) Personal Medical Record*. One by one, all of my healthcare team got a copy and read it. Each one told me that my document helped them quickly focus on me and my problems. Each new team member was provided an up-to-date version. I take a current copy of my medications list to every office visit and a duplicate serves as my checklist when I assemble my medications each week.

My doctor's visits became less complicated. Medical miscommunications became less frequent. But would I have a better chance of surviving my next crisis? It didn't take long to find out.

After some routine blood tests, my brilliant hematologist said, "You're bleeding problem has gotten worse. It's time to act." That led to a discussion with *(My P3A)* who assisted me to prepare for a well-framed, scripted appointment with a faraway subspecialist. Using *My (Unique and Very) Personal Medical Record* and the test results I had brought, the new super-specialist consultant guy was able to efficiently appreciate the history of and the current status of my ailment. A few tests were followed by a new diagnosis — one that pinpointed the cause of my problem. Specific treatment was implemented. This all occurred in one (expensive, time consuming, inconvenient) office visit to my faraway expert. Importantly, my super-specialist confided that my concise, organized, accurate, legible and up-to-date record had enabled him and his team to accomplish in one visit what often takes (expensive, time consuming, inconvenient) weeks and months.

With me as an involved, informed and responsible member, my team of medical professionals has developed a course of treatment. I'm not cured. Perhaps I never will be. But I feel like I have more control over how I'll get where I'm going. I feel safer. I am relieved.

Developing *My (Unique and Very) Personal Medical Record*, providing it to my medical team and chatting from time to time with *(My P3A)* has been time well spent. I observe it has improved my quality of life — and quite possibly has extended my lifespan.

Your personal healthcare journey is bound to be different than mine, but be sure to thoughtfully pack the tools Dr. White has described and have them at your fingertips. They will help you navigate the road ahead.

Bill Theriault
Professor of American Literature
Hagerstown, Maryland

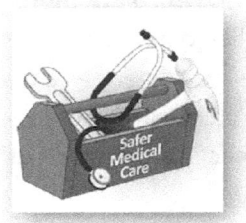

A Senior Physician
Speaks — Steal These Gifts

Much time, energy and financial resources are being spent in the quest for a perfect electronic medical record. Some day that elusive goal will be attained and medical care will be improved immeasurably. At present, however, the systems that exist are far from perfect and often increase rather than decrease the complexity of delivering medical care. As with all things data-driven, the reliability of the output is entirely dependent upon the reliability of the input. Today, in the medical world, the person entering data into a patient's record is often an entry level individual with little medical training. In the days when that data stayed in an office chart, mistakes were not necessarily crucial. Nowadays erroneous information makes its way throughout shared systems and can potentially be much more harmful.

With a full appreciation of the potential shortcomings of the modern healthcare system, Dr. Mike White has provided a powerful antidote in this book, *Safer Medical Care for You and Yours — Six Tools for Safe, Effective Compassionate Care.* From his many years as an educator of physicians and champion for healthcare quality, he has realized the need for every patient to be identified as the unique individual that he or she is. Likewise, that unique individual must help in the creation of an accurate, organized, and up-to-date medical record and keep it at the ready for anticipated and emergent healthcare encounters. In so doing, the individual is positioned to enable and receive the Institute of Medicine's safer, timely, efficient, effective equitable (fair/just) patient-centered medical care.

Not only has Dr. White identified the need for patients to develop and maintain a personal medical record, he has taken the very important next step – he has created the documents to do so. *My (Unique and Very) Personal Medical Record* and *My (Unique and Very) Personal HealthCare Values/Wishes* are priceless gifts from him to anyone who will accept them. One need only download the templates and fill them out.

His prior book, *Safer Medical Care for You and Yours— Four Gifts to Enable Involved, Informed and Responsible Care* contains a number of stories which Dr. White calls charismatic fictions. As a retired surgeon with forty years of experience, I can tell you that these composite stories are not entirely fictitious. They support the need for each of us to develop and maintain a personal medical record. Although I "speak the language," am basically healthy and my care is not complex, a time may arrive when I cannot speak for myself. Therefore, I have personally gone through the process and created *My (Unique and Very) Personal Medical Record* and I do not leave home towards healthcare without it. My document has already proved important and useful to the work of the wonderful teams caring for me and has advanced my care.

I know Dr. White personally as a colleague and friend. I understand his healthcare value (quality, safety and experience) message and I believe I can articulate it — "please steal his gifts, *My (Unique and Very) Personal Medical Record* and *My (Unique and Very) Personal HealthCare Values/Wishes*, emulate them and thereby position you and yours to enable and receive safe and effective compassionate care." If it feels a bit daunting, identify and ask an advocate for assistance. Then, as a favor to Dr. White, me and all those yet to benefit please pass the gifts forward.

Edward J Drawbaugh MD
Director Surgical Services
Hagerstown, Maryland

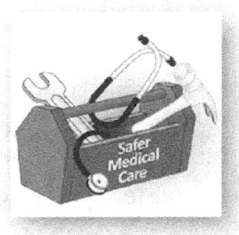

A More Complete Physician

Thinking about, writing about and, actualizing my own preparedness for healthcare I now get it. I have become a more complete physician. I now understand, I was, while well-intentioned, telling patients and families they must go off and accomplish complex and highly emotional tasks when I should have been helping them understand how I might (with all my professional wisdom and experience) personally go about it — that is, share my documents with them. So I have. With mine in hand, they are off and running towards their own unique and very personal records, values and wishes. Their feedback rolls in. They convey that they now get the importance of all of this and in understanding my example they convey:

- *I am now motivated to put my organized and accurate medical record in order and keep it at my fingertips;*
- *I am now, finally, in touch with my own unique and very personal values and wishes;*
- *I have now found my own unique and very personal words and committed them to writing;*
- *I have shared them with my ever so carefully chosen HealthCare Power of Attorney;*
- *He/she has clarified in her/his mind my wishes;*
- *He/she is ready to speak on my behalf should I lose the capacity to speak for myself; and*
- *Most Important #1: I have found peace and tranquility in getting in touch with my values and wishes; and*
- *Most Important #2: my HealthCare Power of Attorney (my near and dear; my significant other; my spouse, my son or daughter) and my personal physicians are all relieved I have this in order.*

Although I anticipated this feedback, I am gratified and buoyed by it.

There was a Most Important #3, that I did not see coming. I have come to understand that after terminal crisis, surviving healthcare powers of attorney — the surviving near and dear — experienced less depression and a better quality of life when their difficult decisions were based upon well-articulated wishes.

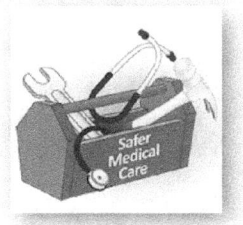

Closure

Back to the beginning — the Institute of Medicine has put forward a well-conceived and clearly articulated national goal — for each individual to be provided healthcare that is safe, timely, efficient, effective equitable and patient-centered (STEEEP). Provided my training and experience, I emphatically concur with and endorse the Institute of Medicine's logic and goal.

The purpose of this concise brochure is to position each unique individual — you, me and those near and dear to us — to enable the better angels assembled to care for us to provide us with safe, effective compassionate care.

This brochure accomplishes this by providing examples of six gift tools for the individual to understand, appreciate and then emulate in her/his uniquely personal manner:

1. My (Unique and Very) Personal Medical Record
2. My Chief Complaint (my story — why I am here today)
3. My (Unique and Very) Personal HealthCare Values/Wishes
4. My HealthCare Power of Attorney and My Advanced Directives
5. My Personal Professional Patient Advocate (My P3A)
6. My Safer Medical Care Emergency Alert System

These tools provide the peace and tranquility associated with confidence that your care will be safe and effective and your unique and very personal values and wishes will be honored should complex healthcare circumstances arise.

Thank you for considering my message. Thank you to Dr. Hightower for amplifying my message with your masterful insights.

I labor daily on a steep learning curve. I anticipate your personal perceptions will assist me to better aid others find safe, effective compassionate care. Should you desire to share your experiences and insights with me, I will be pleased to hear from you. My contact information is as follows:

drmikewhite@tmichaelwhitemd.com or safermedcare@gmail.com
www.tmichaelwhitemd.com or www.safermedcare.com

Respectfully submitted,
Dr. Mike White

Dr. Stephen Hightower Comments

We have put in the work and we deserve to celebrate ourselves for the effort.

May you live long and prosper with your Unique and Very Personal Medical Record, your Health Care Power(s) of Attorney, your Advanced Directives and perhaps your Creative Personal Calling Card at your fingertips.

Respectfully submitted,

Dr. Stephen Hightower

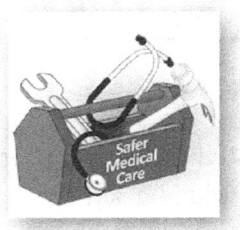

Dr. Hightower's Bio

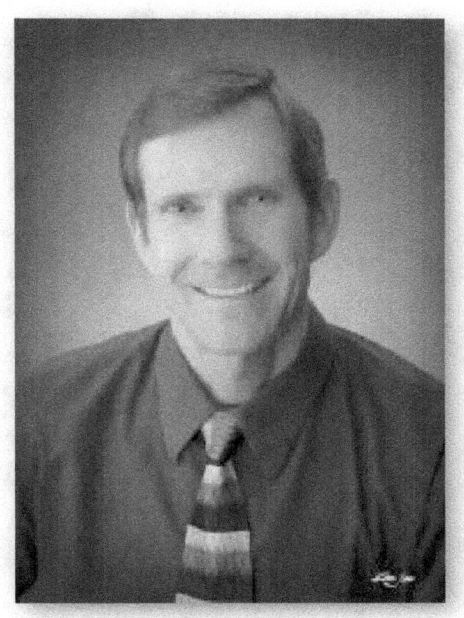

Stephen F Hightower MD FACP is a practicing board-certified specialist in Internal Medicine and Geriatrics. He has worked for over 35 years caring for patients in various environments including the Public Health Service (Truth or Consequences, New Mexico); a community based/university affiliated internal medicine residency program (Johnstown Pennsylvania's Conemaugh Memorial Medical Center); and multispecialty integrated health systems: Baylor/Scott and White (Georgetown, Texas) and Presbyterian Health Care (Albuquerque, New Mexico).

He has served in multiple roles over the years supporting his local medical colleagues including: Chief of Staff (Public Health Service); Associate Residency Program Director (Conemaugh): Champion of the Patient Centered Medical Home Project (Baylor/Scott and White); Lead Physician Internal Medicine (Presbyterian) and medical student faculty and mentor at all institutions.

Dr. Hightower's emphasis for over three decades has been, through empathetic listening and counseling and education, to motivate patients to discover physical and mental lifestyle habits that enable lives well lived.

In *Safer Medical Care for You and Yours — Six Tools for Safe, Effective Compassionate Care*, Dr. Hightower partners with Dr. Mike White to avidly encourage patients to be involved in, informed about and responsible for their healthcare and, in the process, enable safer, effective and compassionate care if/when illness or injury force them to interact with unfamiliar health care systems.

Dr. Hightower lives in Albuquerque, NM with his wife Terri — yes of course, she is a nurse. In their own search for lives well lived, they enjoy bicycling (hills/mountains preferred), visiting the national parks, listening to classical music, and reading about real people who overcome incredible obstacles to succeed (for example, *The Boys in the Boat and Band of Brothers*). Their four grown children are each successfully striving to make positive impacts in their worlds.

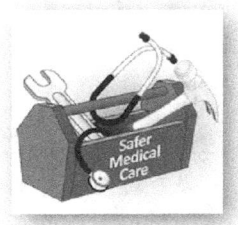

Dr. White's Bio

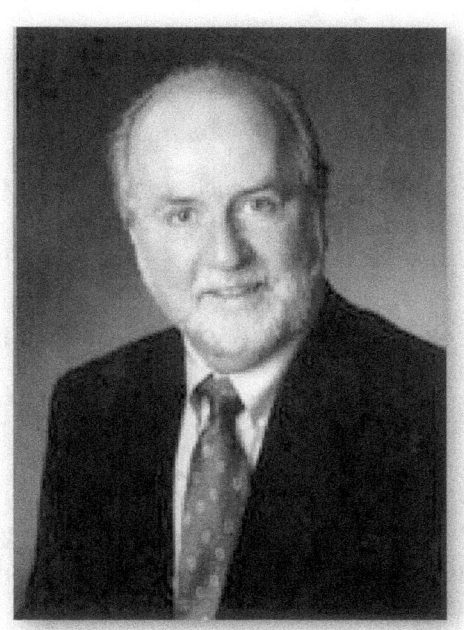

T Michael (Mike) White MD FACP is a HealthCare Value Professional. As a board-certified internist, his general internal medicine career has provided him with experience and insights as a physician: in training, in private practice, faculty member, residency program director (training family medicine, internal medicine, pediatrics, physiatry and psychiatry residents), vice president for value (quality, patient safety, customer satisfaction and profes-sional vitality balanced by cost), vice president for continuing and graduate medical education and healthcare executive (department chair, vice president medical affairs and chief medical officer). In addition, he has the experience and in-sights of a hospital surveyor for The Joint Commission and a field representative for the Accreditation Council Graduate Medical Education's (ACGME) Clinical Learning Environment Review (CLER) Program. Most importantly, Dr. White observes his experiences as a patient have made him a more complete physician.

Dr. White's career has been dedicated to:

- Partnering (through efforts such as this book) with healthcare professionals, patients, families and near and dear significant others to ensure safer, timely, efficient, effective equitable/ just patient-centered medical (STEEEP) care for each intricate and vulnerable individual by enabling each to create her/his own organized and accurate unique and very personal medical record and have it at her/his fingertips,

- Partnering with hospital board, senior executive and medical, nursing, pharmacy, support and therapy staff leadership to advance HealthCare Value. Dr. White equates Health Care Value to compassionate patient care; quality outcomes; patient and staff safety; patient, family and community satisfaction; patient advocacy; and professional vitality balanced by resource utilization/cost and
- Incorporating HealthCare Value concepts into the training of interns, residents and fellows — the preparation of our physicians-in-training as both specialists in their chosen fields and members and leaders of the inter-professional and inter-departmental teams required to efficiently and effectively care for our increasingly intricate and vulnerable patients. Dr. White's formula for realizing resident and fellow proficiency in HealthCare Value has them join, as equal partners, with board, senior executive, graduate medical education, medical staff, nursing, pharmacy and quality/safety leadership in designing, implementing and maintaining the continuously improving systems required to provide safer medical care to the increasingly complex and vulnerable patients and communities our hospitals are privileged to serve.

Dr. White has written and published four books:

- *Unsafe to Safe — An Impatient Proposal for Safe Patient-centered Care* (Amazon; Kindle);
- *A Crystal Spring Thanksgiving — A Little Girl Plays Manly Golf* (Amazon; Kindle);
- *Safer Medical Care for You and Yours — Four Gifts to Enable Involved, Informed and Responsible Care* (Amazon; Kindle); and
- *Safer Medical Care for You and Yours — Six Tools for Safe, Effective Compassionate Care* (Amazon and Kindle).

A fifth book — working title, *A Hub City Murder Mystery* — is in progress.

Beyond the daily study of medicine and his writing, Dr. White enjoys selectively negotiating the New York Times, competitive golf, competitive poker, history, music, cinema, Adirondack boating (Lake George) and thoroughbred racing (Saratoga). He resides with his wife Jacquelyn Forsythe White RN BSN in Hagerstown, Maryland. As he continuously aspires to improve healthcare and a life well-lived, he will be pleased to hear from you at *drmikewhite@tmichaelwhitemd. com* or *safermedcare@gmail.com*.

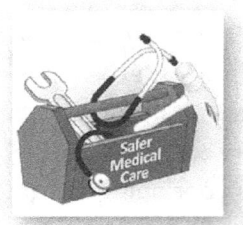

Praise for *Safer Medical Care for You and Yours*

A HealthCare Roadmap

n *Safer Medical Care for You and Yours*, Dr. Mike White has given us a roadmap to navigate the complex and often daunting health care system. As physician caregivers, we all strive to deliver patient-centered care. Without the kind of detailed information provided in *My (Unique and Very Personal) Medical Record* this is very difficult to accomplish in today's busy medical offices and emergency rooms.

Dr. White (a graduate of my Greenwich Hospital/Yale residency) goes well beyond one's personal medical record and delves into personal health care values and wishes and advanced directives. His innovative concept — *My Personal Professional Patient Advocate (My P3A)* — provides a partner to serve as a sounding board for my future important health care decisions. This concept has a unique and important place in medical care.

Dr. White has asked Dr. Stephen Hightower (a graduate of my Phoenix Good Samaritan/Veterans Hospital residency), a distinguished geriatrician, to insert comments as his message unfolds. Their work in tandem is brilliant. I applaud them for collaborating on this important addition to the medical literature.

James L Bernene MD MACP
NCH HealthCare
Naples, Florida

Involved, Informed and Responsible

This is an excellent work. It is definitely an invaluable resource for healthcare providers of all disciplines seeking to provide patient-centered service delivery with optimal quality and high reliability that is visible and transparent to our patients and their families. This is a vital step in the critical pathway towards "broader access to accurate patient information" and dovetails well with national EHR requirements such as ICD 10. More importantly, it is also a must read for individuals who, like you and me, are current or future consumers of healthcare and/or responsible for the healthcare of their loved ones. The time has come for each of us to be involved in, informed about and responsible for our healthcare and position ourselves to receive safe and effective medical care.

Emeric Palmer MD FACP FHM
Hospital Medicine and Hyperbaric Medicine
Consultant in Healthcare IT
Consultant in Physician Documentation
Centreville, Virginia

Crucial Informed Decisions

Safer Medical Care for You and Yours is the discussion a matriarch or patriarch who understands our healthcare system must have with the family. The doctor part of my brain says, "Thank you, Dr. Mike White, for saying so eloquently and precisely what every person in the USA needs to know about our healthcare system." The father part of my brain says, "This is exactly what I need to tell my loved ones about going to a hospital or a doctor's office." The myth in American Healthcare is that there is some doctor or nurse out there ready to take charge of my health and my care. The truth is, for all but a fortunate few of us, that person is me. My healthcare is like my bank account – if I don't manage it, watch out for problems, follow it closely, etc., sooner or later, I'll be in trouble. Investment advisors, stockbrokers, insurance salesmen, accountants, friends and neighbors are all willing to offer advice and help, but at the end of the day, if I don't manage my account, no one else will. The gift, *My (Unique and Very) Personal Medical Record*, is like a bank statement. It is an essential tool that I need to manage my healthcare account. Expert doctors and nurses will certainly find it helpful and will do a better job because it is available to them, but the person it will help the most is me as I take ownership of my health and, in partnership with these experts and my own personal patent advocate (My P3A), make crucial informed decisions about my healthcare.

Dana Kellis MD PhD
Chief Medical Officer, Baptist Health
San Antonio, Texas

A Real Contribution

This professional and artistic work is a real contribution to healthcare value (care, quality, safety and cost). As a golfer to golfers, amateur or pro, *Safer Medical Care for You and Yours* hits healthcare's greens in regulation and comes in under par. What clubs and techniques does Dr. Mike White use to achieve this score? Read this book. The gift tools are there for the taking. Then tweak your own swing and achieve personal health and wellness.

Loren H Roth MD MPH
Associate Senior Vice Chancellor
Clinical Policy, Planning and Health Sciences
University of Pittsburgh

Achieving the Triple Aim

In *Safer Medical Care for You and Yours*, Dr. Mike White encapsulates the ideal state of how a comprehensive medical record looks when it is conscientiously completed. If this were truly taken seriously at the societal level, it would have tremendous benefits to patients, family members and providers alike in achieving "The Triple Aim" of improved quality and patient experience at a lower cost. Tool 3 — *My (Unique and Very) Personal HealthCare Values/Wishes* — in particular is very powerful and important. I see it as dovetailing quite nicely with Atul Gawande's latest work, *"Being Mortal."* Dr. White's contribution has the potential to be one of the best things that medicine has ever done. I hope medicine fully appreciates what he is trying to change.

Brian D Wong MD MPH
Head Coach/CEO, The Bedside Trust
Author, Heroes Need Not Apply

Humane and Favorable Outcomes

Dr. Mike White's outstanding experience and fund of medical knowledge shine through on every page of *Safer Medical Care for You and Yours* — a fine addition to the medical safety canon. No one except the late Oliver Saks MD writes as feelingly and perceptively about case studies. Dr. White compellingly shows how handy (at one's fingertips) personal medical records save lives and how My Personal Professional Patient Advocates (My P3As) steer care away from callous courses and towards humane and favorable outcomes. I hope this slim and deeply meaningful volume finds its way into the hands of patients and providers alike.

Attorney James Lieber
Author, Killer Care
Pittsburgh, Pennsylvania

A Must Do

As one who has used Dr. White as a *My Personal Professional Patient Advocate (My P3A)*, I attest to and join Dr. White's righteous fervor for his development and implementation of the essential instrument — *My (Unique and Very) Personal Medical Record*. The process has made me a more involved, informed and responsible patient and has benefited me and those that care for and about me. *Safer Medical Care for You and Yours* is exceptionally well done and makes an engaging case for the thoughtful ninety minute construction of one's own organized, accurate and up-to date very personal medical record.

Carl Galligan PhD
Dean Emeritus
Hagerstown Community College

Patient — the Nucleus of Healthcare

Patient safety concerns have forced healthcare to digitalize and standardize, often at the expense of the patient. While providing for safer and more consistent care, person-centered care has been compromised. The six tools gifted in *Safer Medical Care for You and Yours* provide the solution patients, families and providers are seeking to restore the patient as the nucleus of healthcare. Dr. Mike White gives back to healthcare the gift of a patient-centric, laser focused clinical dynamic that creates the foundation for a safer, more efficient and more effective healthcare encounter for both patients and providers.

Ellen Amalfitano RN PhD
Director, Performance Partners
Premier, Inc.

A Masterful Tool

The medical community is truly lucky to have someone like Dr. Mike White take on the subject of patient safety in general and medical care guidelines in particular. Both physicians and patients and their families have struggled with the issue for decades. We have witnessed occasions when two or more providers speak with a patient or a family member and come out with different sets of instructions. Neither the medical providers nor the public are well educated on the matter. No one masters the capacity to bridge this gap better than Dr. White. This book is a great tool for medical providers and patients alike.

Ibrahim Ghobrial MD FACP
Program Director, Internal Medicine Residency
UPMC McKeesport

Prepared and Decisive

These tools are meaningful and excellent. Unfortunately, the sickest, most complicated people will be the least likely to use them. There remains the attitude in the majority of people that "the doctor always knows best" and they just trust in her/him and the medical team to do right by them.

As a senior nurse, I always advocated for my patients, but I dare say that this next generation does not spend as much time or attention on their patients to be their advocates. They do not have time and have not been trained to advocate. Therefore, each individual (you and me) must.

It really does help to have a medical person to be an advocate — not everyone is so lucky to know one that they can ask. Even with that, you have to be prepared and decisive. *Safer Medical Care* provides the tools.

Ms. Jackie Gormly RN
Rutland, Vermont

Optimum Care

As a Registered Nurse, who worked in Trauma, ICU and ED, I love this book!! So many times, I experienced patients arriving without the ability to talk. The lifesaving team always searched for identification and information — we searched in the wallet, the purse, the pockets, anywhere a patient might have information regarding allergies, medications and conditions. Too often we initiated care without knowing if a medicine or treatment would help or harm the patient. Sometimes, we withheld a medicine or treatment until we could ascertain the patient's history because the thing that would do the most for them might be the worst for them.

Dr. White's book is a powerful resource for all medical personnel both for lifesaving situations and also to optimize care for a patient seeking care from a specialist. Unless you have been fortunate to have the same physician for 40 years, and you have never seen any other physicians, the simple tool described in the book will help your medical team optimize your care. Even if you have only seen that one physician your entire life, if you are ever injured or need to seek care elsewhere you will need the tool described in this book to help your medical professionals care for you.

This is an awesome book. I have used the tool when seeing my own specialist. It helped him spend more time with me and less time trying to put the pieces together of my medical history. Because even I was rather nervous, and my medical history is only as good as my ability to remember my 66 years of medical care, the information provided to my specialist physician was essential to allow him to diagnose my problem and help me find a solution. Over 60% of the information a team uses to determine a diagnosis and treatment plan comes from the history the patient provides.

I highly recommend Dr. White's book to you and those you love. It could save your life.

Ms. Mary Towe BSN MBA
Hagerstown, Maryland

Especially Prudent

As a practicing clinical pharmaceutical specialist, I am well aware of the risks associated with healthcare delivery. Errors can and do result from a lack of pertinent information. In this regard, it seems simply common sense that an all-encompassing, up-to-date, body of knowledge which speaks to one's (yours or your loved ones) healthcare conditions and procedures, desires, ethical philosophies and spiritual needs, accompany the individual into the healthcare arena. This is especially prudent in times when an individual is most vulnerable and potentially unable to speak out for themselves.

In *Safer Medical Care for You and Yours*, T Michael White, MD, comprehensively outlines an approach and provides documentation tools which allow you to customize a detailed menu of care for yourself and/or your family members. Effectively outlining your specific conditions of health and how you wish your medical team and family to proceed in the unfortunate event that you are unable to steer your own path.

I have my own tragic missed opportunity — after my father suffered a devastating intracranial bleed, he lay slowly deteriorating in a nursing home bed for many months, unable to communicate clearly. My father's second wife (a woman with mixed incentives) took it upon herself to exclude me from any and all decision-making with respect to his care. Living out of state at the time, she managed to conceal his passing from me, successfully preventing me from being able to say goodbye to him before he died.

Dr. White's guidelines should prevent such a pitifully painful situation. I will heed the good doctor's advice and assure that my healthcare conditions and desires are communicated precisely and in timely fashion to my healthcare team, regardless of how "bullet-proof" I currently feel. Thank you Dr. White. It is my hope that all who read your words embrace the approaches you have so eloquently described!

C W Fetrow PharmD
West Palm Beach, Florida

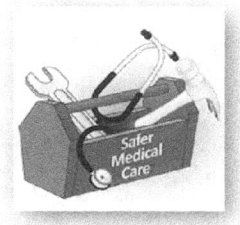

NOTES

Wallet Card
(for copying and personalizing)

IN EMERGENCY SEE REVERSE

Safer Medical Care

W   E

S

Safer Medical Care for You and Yours • www.tmichaelwhitemd.com

IN EMERGENCY CALL

Phone #: _____

or

Phone #: _____

for

My (Unique and Very) Personal Medical Record

www.ingramcontent.com/pod-product-compliance
Lightning Source LLC
Chambersburg PA
CBHW081851280526

45789CB00007B/2654